Gut Health Made Easy for Women over 40

Recipes to Revitalize Your Body and Mind, Manage Menopause Symptoms, Balance Hormones, and Lose Weight with Delicious Smoothies, Salads, and Soups

Lara West

First edition

Contents

1

Introduction

Dear girlfriend, I am so thrilled to embark on a culinary adventure with you and to dive into a world of flavors, nourishment, and vibrant well-being!

This cookbook is the perfect companion for the transformation you experienced after reading my first book *"7 Healthy Gut Habits for Women Over 40: Get Your Life Back Using Intermittent Fasting, Nutrition, and Self-Care to Restore Gut Microbiome for Weight Loss and Increased Energy."*

It isn't just a compilation of recipes; it's a heartfelt invitation to explore the incredible potential of nourishing foods and their transformative impact on our lives. As women navigating the enriching journey of life over 40, our bodies deserve the utmost care and nourishment. With this in mind, I've poured my heart into crafting these recipes, each one designed to empower you to take control of your gut health and navigate menopause symptoms with more ease.

There's something that compelled me to create this cookbook—the feedback I received from remarkable women who read my first book. Many shared their journey with me, expressing a desire for wholesome recipes that align with their wellness goals. They mentioned feeling a gap in their meal plans and asked if I could share the nourishing meals I prepare. These conversations and shared experiences breathed life into this collection of recipes.

We will be building upon the solid foundation we laid in that book and taking our gut health game to a whole new level of deliciousness.

In case you haven't had the chance to read my first book, I included the Amazon link at the end, together with the link to download the companion workbook. But for now, let me give you a brief recap of those 7 powerful, healthy gut habits. These habits are the building blocks of well-being, the secret sauce that has helped me and countless women manage menopause symptoms and reclaim their vitality.

1. Habit One: Skip a Meal

Intermittent fasting has proven to be a game-changer in supporting hormonal balance, weight management, and gut health. By allowing our bodies to experience periods of fasting, we promote cellular repair and metabolic flexibility and optimize the intricate dance of our hormones.

2. Habit Two: Make Biotics Your Friends

Prebiotics and probiotics are our allies in cultivating a thriving gut microbiome. By incorporating prebiotic and probiotic-rich food into our diets, we nourish the beneficial bacteria that support our immune function, digestion, and overall gut health.

3. Habit Three: Count Your Chews

Mindful eating is a powerful practice that creates a deeper connection between our bodies and the food we consume. By slowing down, savoring each bite, and paying attention to our body's cues, we improve digestion, enhance nutrient absorption, and foster a healthier relationship with food.

4. Habit Four: Read the Labels

Understanding the impact of our food choices is crucial for nurturing our gut health. By avoiding processed foods, excessive sugar, unhealthy fats, and external toxins found in our cosmetics and cleaning products, we empower ourselves to make informed choices that support our well-being.

5. Habit Five: Get Up and Move

Exercise is not just about maintaining a healthy weight; it plays a vital role in gut health as well. Physical activity boosts digestion, reduces inflammation, and improves the composition of the gut microbiome. Lace up those sneakers and celebrate the joy of movement!

6. Habit Six: Catch Enough ZZZ's

Sleep is a cornerstone of optimal health, and it has a significant impact on our gut health. By prioritizing restful sleep and adopting healthy sleep habits, we support our gut-brain connection, promote hormonal balance, and improve cognitive function.

7. Habit Seven: Take a Breather

Managing stress is essential for our gut health journey. Incorporating stress management techniques such as meditation, journaling, and embracing the cozy concept of Hygge allows us to unwind, reduce inflammation, and cultivate a sense of calm amid life's challenges.

These 7 healthy gut habits have transformed lives and continue to do so. If you haven't had the chance to explore my first book, I encourage you to read it, absorb the knowledge, and start implementing these habits. It's never too late to embark on a path of vibrant health and manage menopause symptoms with grace and resilience.

I developed these healthy habits because, just like you, I faced many health challenges when I hit the milestone age of 40. As I started experiencing perimenopause symptoms, I was also diagnosed with leaky gut syndrome and an autoimmune disease. It was a difficult time, but it was also a time of self-discovery, a deep dive into learning the world of gut health, adopting new habits, and exploring the remarkable power of cooking nourishing meals. This journey unlocked the secrets to vibrant wellness and revealed the incredible potential of food as a source of healing. Through my own struggles, I discovered the powerful connection between gut health, perimenopause and menopause symptoms, self-care, and healthy lifestyle habits. I also discovered the joy of preparing delicious, nourishing meals.

But let's start with the fascinating realm of our gut microbiome—the ecosystem of microorganisms that live in our digestive tract. Within this bustling metropolis, trillions of microscopic inhabitants, including bacteria, viruses, fungi, and other microbes, coexist in a delicate balance. These remarkable organisms play a fundamental role in our health, exerting a profound influence on various aspects of our well-being.

The gut microbiome is often referred to as our "second brain" because of its extensive communication network with our central nervous system. It produces an array of neurotransmitters and chemical messengers that can influence our mood, cognition, and behavior. Our gut microbiome is intricately involved in our immune system's function, playing a crucial role in defending against harmful pathogens and promoting a balanced inflammatory response.

In menopause, the gut microbiome takes on even greater significance. Research has revealed a fascinating connection between the gut microbiome and the hormonal changes that occur during this transformative stage of life. As our bodies transition through menopause, fluctuations in hormone levels can disrupt the balance of our gut microbiome, leading to a cascade of symptoms that may catch us off-guard.

Hormonal changes affecting our gut microbiome are often the reason for hot flashes, sudden waves of heat that wash over our bodies. The interplay between our hormones and gut microbes may also influence sleep disturbances, another common menopause symptom. Fluctuations in estrogen levels can affect our gut microbiome, leading to imbalances that contribute to mood swings, brain fog, and weight gain.

Understanding this relationship between the gut microbiome and menopause symptoms is key to unlocking the potential for managing these challenges and promoting overall well-being. By nourishing our gut microbiome through a diet rich in whole foods, we can cultivate a thriving ecosystem within, supporting hormonal balance, enhancing immune function, and managing the troublesome symptoms that often accompany this stage of life.

This book will guide you on a path of rejuvenation and empowerment. We will explore a variety of delicious recipes designed to nourish and support our gut. I crafted these recipes to incorporate gut-healthy ingredients such as fiber-rich foods, prebiotics, probiotics, omega-3 fatty acids, and antioxidants. By incorporating these gut-healthy foods into our meals, we provide the essential nutrients and beneficial compounds that support a flourishing gut microbiome, helping us navigate the challenges of menopause with greater ease. Through the power of food, we will restore balance, enhance our vitality, and reclaim our sense of well-being.

Now, I'd like to be candid with you. I'm not a professional cook, so these recipes may not be perfect and can certainly be improved. I'm here to learn and grow just like you, and your feedback is invaluable to making these recipes even better. Calculating nutritional values isn't my expertise either, but what I can assure you is that these recipes are filled with wholesome ingredients that can make a positive impact on your health. And I apologize for not including photos—it would have taken ages, and my priority was to get this book to you as quickly as possible. The recipes and the nourishing value they offer are what matter most. And remember, portion sizes may vary depending on your individual weight loss goals, so don't hesitate to tailor these recipes to your needs.

As we stand at the threshold of this culinary journey, let's dive into the heart of the matter – the essential building blocks of nourishment. In the first chapter, we'll unravel the remarkable benefits that lie within different food groups, understanding how each contributes to our gut health, hormonal balance, and overall vitality.

2

Fueling and Healing the Gut: Food Groups

Fiber-Rich Foods

Let's begin our journey toward a healthy gut with an understanding of the importance of dietary fiber. Fiber is a type of carbohydrate that our body cannot digest fully, passing through the digestive tract relatively intact. While it may seem unassuming, fiber plays a crucial role in promoting gut health and overall well-being.

Consuming an adequate amount of dietary fiber has many benefits for our gut health. First, fiber provides nourishment to the beneficial bacteria living in our gut. These bacteria ferment fiber, producing short-chain fatty acids (SCFAs) as byproducts. SCFAs, such as butyrate, propionate, and acetate, have anti-inflammatory properties, provide energy to the cells, and help maintain a healthy gut environment.

Fiber helps regulate bowel movements and prevent constipation by adding bulk to the stool and promoting regularity. It also aids in weight management by promoting a feeling of fullness, preventing overeating, and supporting healthy digestion.

One crucial role of fiber is its ability to stimulate the production of mucus in the gut, which plays a vital role in fortifying the gut's protective barrier. The mucous layer acts as a physical barrier, shielding the delicate lining of the intestines from harmful bacteria and irritants. By promoting the production of mucus, fiber helps maintain the integrity of this protective barrier, reducing the risk of inflammation and damage to the gut lining. The mucous layer serves as a nourishing environment for beneficial bacteria in the gut, allowing them to thrive and carry out their essential functions.

Studies have also shown that a fiber-rich diet is associated with a reduced risk of various chronic diseases, including heart disease, type 2 diabetes, and certain types of cancer. The protective effects of fiber can be attributed, in part, to its role in maintaining a healthy gut microbiome and modulating inflammation in the body. [1]

High-fiber food sources

To incorporate more fiber into your diet, focus on consuming a variety of plant-based foods. Here are some excellent sources of dietary fiber:

Whole Grains

Fruits and vegetables

Legumes

Nuts and seeds

Psyllium husk

Whole Grains. Opt for whole grain products such as brown rice, quinoa, whole wheat, and oatmeal. These grains keep their bran and germ, which are rich in fiber.

Fruits and vegetables. Include a wide range of fruits and vegetables in your meals. Berries, apples, pears, oranges, broccoli, Brussels sprouts, carrots, and leafy greens like spinach and kale are especially high in fiber.

Legumes. Beans, lentils, chickpeas, and other legumes are not only rich in fiber but also provide valuable plant-based protein. Add them to soups, stews, and salads, or enjoy them as a main dish.

Nuts and seeds. Almonds, chia seeds, flaxseeds, and pumpkin seeds are fiber-packed snacks that can be enjoyed on their own or added to yogurt, smoothies, or salads.

Psyllium husk. Psyllium husk is a soluble fiber supplement that can be added to smoothies or mixed with water for an easy way to boost your fiber intake.

If your diet is low in fiber, remember to increase your fiber intake gradually and drink plenty of water to aid in digestion and prevent any discomfort associated with sudden changes in dietary fiber. This helps fiber move smoothly through your digestive system and promotes optimal gut function.

By incorporating fiber-rich foods into your diet, you'll nourish your gut microbiome, promote healthy digestion, and support overall gut health. [2]

The Impact of Gluten and GMO Crops on the Gut

In recent years, gluten intolerance has become a significant consideration for gut health. Gluten is a protein found in wheat, barley, and rye, i.e. grains rich in fiber. However, it can trigger adverse reactions in individuals with gluten intolerance or celiac disease. These conditions can lead to gut inflammation, digestive discomfort, and other symptoms that compromise overall well-being. For those with gluten intolerance or celiac disease, adopting a gluten-free diet is crucial for gut health and overall health. [3]

If this is you, focus on whole foods like fruits, vegetables, legumes, and naturally gluten-free grains such as quinoa, millet, buckwheat, amaranth, tapioca (cassava root), arrowroot, sorghum, and brown rice. Read food labels carefully to identify hidden sources of gluten and seek gluten-free alternatives. If you suspect gluten intolerance, consulting with a healthcare professional or a registered dietitian will provide personalized guidance on managing it.

The cultivation of genetically modified crops (GMO) has raised concerns about their potential impact on gut health. GMO crops are modified to be resistant to pests or herbicides, and their widespread use has led to increased exposure to chemical residues. Research on the long-term effects of GMOs on the gut is ongoing, and some studies suggest disruptions to the gut microbiome and increased inflammation.

To minimize exposure to GMOs and potential gut health concerns, consider choosing organic products whenever possible. Organic foods are grown without genetically modified ingredients and pesticides and are produced using methods that prioritize environmental sustainability and the well-being of both consumers and the ecosystem. Look for the USDA (or your country's) organic seal on food packaging, which ensures that the product meets strict organic standards.

By being mindful of gluten intake and opting for organic products, you can support a gut-healthy lifestyle and make choices that align with your well-being goals.

Prebiotics

Prebiotics are like fuel for the friendly bacteria in your gut. They offer many benefits that can support your gut health.

One of the key advantages of prebiotics is their ability to promote the growth of beneficial bacteria in your gut. They help with digestion, enhance nutrient absorption, and support your immune function.

Another significant benefit of prebiotics is their role in fortifying your gut's protective barrier, as described in the previous section about fiber. A lot of fiber-rich foods are also rich in prebiotics. They stimulate the production of mucus in your intestinal lining, which acts as a shield against harmful substances. By strengthening this barrier, prebiotics help defend against pathogens and reduce the risk of gut-related issues.

If you've been struggling with irregular bowel movements, prebiotics can help regulate them. They contribute to the overall balance and efficiency of your digestive system, promoting bowel regularity and reducing the likelihood of constipation.

Prebiotics may also play a role in weight management. They can make you feel fuller for longer, reducing your calorie intake and helping you maintain a healthy weight. Prebiotics have also been linked to potential anti-inflammatory effects, which can help reduce systemic inflammation in your body.

One notable advantage of prebiotics is their ability to improve the absorption of several essential minerals. Prebiotics, particularly soluble fibers like inulin and oligofructose (a subgroup of inulin), act as carriers for minerals such as calcium, magnesium, and iron, helping enhance their bio-availability. By improving mineral absorption, prebiotics help maintain healthy bones, optimal nerve function, and prevent nutrient deficiencies.

Prebiotics have also been associated with the potential benefit of lowering cholesterol levels. Certain types of prebiotics, like beta-glucans found in oats and barley, have been shown to have cholesterol-lowering effects. These prebiotics bind to cholesterol in the gut, preventing its absorption into the bloodstream. As a result, consuming prebiotic-rich foods may help reduce LDL (bad) cholesterol levels and improve heart health. [4].

Prebiotic Food Sources

Including prebiotic-rich foods in your daily meals is a practical way to support your gut health. Here are some examples of prebiotic food sources:

Chicory Root

Garlic, Leeks, and Onions

Asparagus

Bananas

Legumes

Whole Grains

Jerusalem Artichokes

Dandelion Greens

Cocoa

Apples

Flaxseeds

Yakon Root

Jicama Root

Seaweed

Yams

Sweet potatoes (all kinds)

Carrots

Celery

Probiotics and Fermented Foods

Probiotics play a vital role in promoting a healthy gut. Probiotics are live microorganisms that, when consumed in adequate amounts, offer many health benefits for the gut.

One of the key benefits of probiotics is their ability to restore and maintain a healthy balance of gut bacteria. Factors such as stress, poor diet, antibiotics, and aging can disrupt the natural equilibrium of our gut microbiome. This imbalance, known as dysbiosis, can lead to digestive issues, compromised immune function, and other health problems. By introducing probiotics into our diet, we can replenish and diversify the beneficial bacteria in our gut, fostering a healthier microbial community.

Research has shown that probiotics can aid in the digestion and absorption of nutrients, improve bowel regularity, and enhance overall gut function. These beneficial bacteria produce enzymes that help break down complex carbohydrates, fibers, and proteins, making them more accessible for our bodies to absorb and use. As a result, consuming probiotic-rich foods can optimize nutrient absorption and promote better digestive health.

Probiotics exert various effects on the immune system. They interact with immune cells in the gut, stimulating the production of protective substances and promoting a balanced immune response. By supporting immune function in the gut, probiotics contribute to the overall well-being of our immune system, which plays a crucial role in defending against harmful pathogens and maintaining good health.

Incorporating probiotic-rich foods into your diet is an excellent way to boost your gut health. Fermented foods, in particular, are a wonderful source of probiotics. Fermentation is a natural process in which beneficial bacteria convert sugars and carbohydrates into lactic acid, creating an acidic environment that inhibits the growth of harmful bacteria. This process enhances the shelf life of the food and increases its nutritional value. By consuming fermented foods, we introduce live probiotic cultures into our digestive system, positively affecting our gut microbiome. [5].

Probiotic and Fermented Food Sources

Incorporate probiotic and fermented foods into your diet to enhance your gut health and introduce beneficial bacteria into your system. Here are some examples of probiotic and fermented foods that undergo a natural fermentation process that encourages the growth of beneficial microorganisms, resulting in a rich source of probiotics:

Yogurt

Kefir

Sauerkraut (fermented and refrigerated)

Kimchi

Miso

Tempeh

Kombucha

Kvass

Raw Cheeses

Apple Cider Vinegar

Pickles in Brine (fermented and refrigerated)

Yogurt is one of the most well-known probiotic foods. It is made by fermenting milk with specific strains of bacteria, such as Lactobacillus Bulgaricus and Streptococcus Thermophilus. Look for yogurt labeled with "live and active cultures" with no added sugar to ensure you're getting the beneficial bacteria without extra calories.

Kefir is a fermented milk drink that is rich in probiotics. It is made by combining Kefir grains with milk, which undergoes fermentation. Kefir contains a diverse range of beneficial bacteria and yeasts, offering many potential health benefits for the gut.

Sauerkraut is a fermented cabbage dish that originates from Eastern Europe. It is made by fermenting cabbage with salt, allowing lactic acid bacteria to thrive. Sauerkraut is a good source of probiotics and also provides vitamins C and K. Only look for sauerkraut in a refrigerated section of your supermarket. Sauerkraut with a long shelf life without refrigeration is just salted cabbage and has no beneficial bacteria.

Kimchi is a traditional Korean side dish made from fermented vegetables, typically cabbage and radishes. It is seasoned with spices, garlic, and ginger. Kimchi contains various strains of lactic acid bacteria and is known for its bold and tangy flavors.

Miso is a traditional Japanese seasoning made from fermented soybeans, rice, and barley. It is commonly used in soups and marinades. Miso fermentation involves the action of specific fungi and bacteria, resulting in a rich Umami flavor and probiotic content.

Tempeh is a fermented soy product that originated in Indonesia. It is made by fermenting soybeans with a specific type of fungus. Tempeh is not only a great source of probiotics but also provides plant-based protein and nutrients.

Kombucha is a fermented tea beverage. It is made by fermenting sweetened tea with a symbiotic culture of bacteria and yeast (SCOBY). Kombucha offers a refreshing and tangy taste along with probiotic benefits but you should be mindful of its high sugar content.

Kvass is a beloved traditional fermented beverage that holds a special place in my heart, as it is a popular drink in Ukraine, my home country. This tangy and refreshing elixir is made from fermented rye bread, resulting in a unique flavor. Kvass has been enjoyed for centuries in Eastern Europe and is known for its probiotic properties, thanks to the beneficial lactic acid bacteria that develop during the fermentation process. It's not only a delightful beverage but also a wonderful way to incorporate probiotic-rich foods into your diet, supporting the health and diversity of your gut microbiome.

Raw Cheeses. Certain types of raw cheeses, such as Gouda, cheddar, provolone, Gruyère, Edam, Feta, Parmesan, Swiss, and cottage cheese, undergo natural fermentation processes that result in the development of probiotic cultures. These cheeses provide a savory flavor along with probiotic benefits. Only cheeses that have been aged but not heated have probiotics, so check the labels to make sure you're buying fermented raw cheese and not processed pasteurized cheese.

Apple Cider Vinegar is fermented apple juice. It contains acetic acid and various beneficial bacteria. Including apple cider vinegar in your diet, such as in salad dressings or diluted in water, will contribute to your probiotic intake.

Pickles in Brine. These pickles are made through the traditional fermentation process, using saltwater brine, which offers probiotic benefits. Enjoy these tangy and crunchy pickles as a snack or add them to sandwiches and salads for a flavorful twist. Only buy pickles in the refrigerated section.

Incorporating these probiotic and fermented foods into your diet will contribute to a healthier gut microbiome. Remember to read the labels and choose only unpasteurized and traditionally fermented versions of these foods to ensure the presence of live cultures and probiotics.

Foods Rich in Omega-3

Omega-3 fatty acids play a crucial role in supporting gut health and overall well-being. [6]. These fatty acids, including eicosapentaenoic acid (EPA) and docosahexaenoic acid (DHA), are commonly found in fatty fish, such as salmon, mackerel, and sardines, as well as in plant-based sources like flaxseeds, chia seeds, and walnuts.

One of the key benefits of omega-3 fatty acids for gut health is their anti-inflammatory properties. They help reduce inflammation in the gut by inhibiting the production of pro-inflammatory molecules and promoting the synthesis of anti-inflammatory compounds. By calming inflammation, omega-3 fatty acids can support a healthier gut environment and alleviate symptoms associated with digestive issues.

Omega-3 fatty acids also play a role in maintaining the integrity of the gut lining. They help strengthen and repair the gut lining, enhancing its barrier function and reducing the risk of a leaky gut.

Omega-3 fatty acids also support the growth and diversity of beneficial gut bacteria. They provide nourishment and create an environment that promotes the growth of these bacteria while inhibiting the growth of harmful bacteria. This balance of gut bacteria is essential for proper digestion, nutrient absorption, and immune function.

One notable benefit of omega-3 fatty acids is their ability to help lower "bad" cholesterol levels and reduce high blood pressure. Studies have shown that consuming omega-3-rich foods or supplements can help reduce triglyceride levels in the blood and increase levels of high-density lipoprotein (HDL) cholesterol, commonly known as the "good" cholesterol. This can have a positive impact on cardiovascular health, as elevated levels of LDL cholesterol and high blood pressure are risk factors for heart disease.

Omega-3 fatty acids have been linked to improved cognitive health and a reduced risk of age-related cognitive decline and dementia. The brain highly depends on healthy fats, and omega-3 fatty acids are essential for supporting brain function and structure. Research suggests that omega-3 fatty acids may help protect against cognitive decline, improve memory, and enhance overall brain health. These benefits extend to gut health, as the gut and brain are interconnected through the gut-brain axis, and a healthy gut contributes to optimal brain function.

Besides cardiovascular and cognitive benefits, omega-3 supplementation can help reduce joint pain, stiffness, and swelling in individuals with rheumatoid arthritis, a chronic autoimmune condition characterized by inflammation in the joints. [7]. Omega-3 fatty acids' anti-inflammatory properties can also benefit bone health by reducing inflammation in the bone tissue, supporting bone strength, and reducing the risk of osteoporosis. This becomes very important for us, women, as we experience a higher risk of osteoporosis as we enter menopause due to low estrogen levels.

Omega-3 Food Sources

As you can see, incorporating omega-3 fatty acids into your diet is essential for promoting gut health and overall health, especially after 40. While supplementation is an option, getting these beneficial fats from whole foods is always preferred as they come bundled with other valuable nutrients. [8]

Here are some excellent food sources of omega-3 fatty acids:

Fatty Fish

Flaxseeds

Chia seeds

Walnuts

Hemp seeds

Seaweed

Egg yolks

Fatty Fish. Alaskan salmon, Atlantic mackerel, sardines, trout, herring, anchovies, and Albacore tuna are among the richest sources of omega-3. These fish accumulate high levels of EPA and DHA because they consume algae and other marine microorganisms. Aim to include fatty fish in your diet at least twice a week to reap the benefits of omega-3 fatty acids.

Flaxseeds are a plant-based source of omega-3. They are rich in alpha-linolenic acid (ALA), which is converted into EPA and DHA in the body, although the conversion efficiency is relatively low. Grinding flaxseeds before consumption enhances their digestibility and allows better nutrient absorption. Add ground flaxseeds to smoothies, oatmeal, yogurt, or baked goods to boost your omega-3 intake.

Chia seeds are another plant-based omega-3 powerhouse. They contain a good balance of omega-3, omega-6, and omega-9 fatty acids. These tiny seeds can absorb liquid and form a gel-like consistency, making them a versatile ingredient in puddings, smoothies, or as an egg substitute in baking recipes.

Walnuts are not only a tasty snack but also an excellent source of plant-based omega-3. They contain a significant amount of ALA, making them a valuable addition to a gut-healthy diet. Sprinkle walnuts over salads, incorporate them into homemade granola, or enjoy them as a snack for a satisfying dose of omega-3.

Hemp seeds are a nutritional powerhouse, providing a range of beneficial nutrients. They contain a balanced ratio of omega-3 and omega-6 fatty acids. Add hemp seeds to smoothies, sprinkle them over salads or roasted vegetables, or include them in homemade energy bars for a nutrient boost.

Seaweed is a marine vegetable that is rich in various nutrients, including omega-3 fatty acids. Certain types of seaweed, such as kelp, nori, and wakame, are excellent sources of EPA and DHA. Incorporate seaweed into your diet by enjoying sushi rolls wrapped in nori or adding dried seaweed flakes to soups, salads, or stir-fries.

Egg yolks are a nutritious source of omega-3 fatty acids. While the levels may vary depending on the diet of the hens, eggs from pasture-raised or omega-3-enriched hens have a higher omega-3 content. Include eggs as part of your balanced diet to benefit from their omega-3 content along with other essential nutrients.

Anti-inflammatory Foods and Antioxidants

Inflammation is a natural response by the body's immune system to protect against harmful stimuli such as infection, injury, or toxins. While acute inflammation is essential for healing, chronic inflammation has detrimental effects on gut health and overall well-being.

Chronic inflammation in the gut can disrupt the delicate balance of the gut microbiome, leading to a range of digestive issues and contributing to various health conditions. Inflammatory bowel diseases (IBD), including Crohn's disease and ulcerative colitis, are characterized by chronic inflammation in the digestive tract, resulting in symptoms like abdominal pain, diarrhea, etc.

Research has shown that chronic inflammation in the gut is not limited to gastrointestinal issues alone. It has been linked to systemic inflammation, which can affect other areas of the body, including the cardiovascular system, joints, and even the brain. There is emerging evidence linking chronic gut inflammation to conditions like cardiovascular disease, rheumatoid arthritis, and neurodegenerative diseases such as Alzheimer's and Parkinson's. [9]

The gut plays a crucial role in immune function, nutrient absorption, and overall health. When inflammation disrupts the delicate balance of the gut, it can compromise these functions and contribute to a cascade of health problems. This is why managing inflammation in the gut is vital for maintaining optimal gut health.

Fortunately, by incorporating anti-inflammatory foods into your diet, you can help reduce gut inflammation and support a healthier gut environment. [10]. These foods are rich in compounds that inhibit pro-inflammatory pathways, reduce oxidative stress, and promote gut healing.

Food Sources to Help Reduce Inflammation

Choosing the right foods can make a significant difference in reducing inflammation and promoting a healthy gut. Incorporating these foods into your diet can provide essential nutrients and bioactive compounds that have anti-inflammatory properties.

Here are some of these gut-supportive and anti-inflammatory foods:

Fatty Fish

Berries

Leafy Greens

Turmeric

Cinnamon

Extra Virgin Olive Oil

Nuts and Seeds

Ginger

Broccoli

Avocados

Green Tea

Matcha Green Tea

Cocoa

Mushrooms

Grapes

Tomatoes

Cherries

Goji Berries

Chia Seeds

Hemp Hearts

Pineapple

Citrus Fruits

Incorporating these foods into your diet can provide a wide range of anti-inflammatory compounds, antioxidants, and other beneficial nutrients. We will use them in different recipes and combinations later in the book to enjoy their flavors while reaping the potential health benefits they offer. Remember, variety is key to a balanced and gut-healthy diet.

Essential Vitamins, Minerals, and "Superfoods"

A well-nourished gut relies on a variety of essential nutrients to support its health and optimal functioning. Among these, vitamins and minerals play vital roles in maintaining gut health. Let's explore some key vitamins and minerals and their contributions.

Vitamin A. This nutrient supports the health and integrity of the gut lining. It promotes the production of mucus and enhances the immune response in the gut. Good sources of vitamin A include sweet potatoes, carrots, spinach, and kale. [11]

Vitamin D. Known as the "sunshine vitamin," vitamin D plays a role in modulating immune function and reducing gut inflammation. It also supports the absorption of calcium and phosphorus, contributing to overall bone health. Fatty fish like salmon and mackerel, fortified dairy products, and exposure to sunlight are sources of vitamin D.[12]

Vitamin E. With its antioxidant properties, vitamin E helps protect the gut cells from oxidative damage. It supports immune function and aids in reducing inflammation. Foods rich in vitamin E include almonds, sunflower seeds, spinach, and avocados. [13]

B Vitamins. The B vitamins, including B1 (thiamine), B2 (riboflavin), B3 (niacin), B6, B9 (folate), and B12, play various roles in gut health. They support energy production, promote proper digestion and nutrient absorption, and contribute to the overall health of the gut lining. Whole grains, legumes, leafy greens, and certain animal products (beef, poultry, and fish) are good sources of B vitamins. [14]

Zinc. This mineral is essential for maintaining the integrity of the gut lining and promoting wound healing. It supports the immune system and helps in the production of enzymes involved in digestion. Foods rich in zinc include oysters, beef, poultry, pumpkin seeds, and chickpeas. [15]

Magnesium. Magnesium contributes to muscle relaxation and helps regulate bowel movements, thus supporting healthy digestion. It also plays a role in maintaining the gut barrier function and reducing inflammation. Leafy greens, nuts, seeds, and whole grains are good sources of magnesium. [16]

Selenium. Selenium is an antioxidant mineral that supports gut health by protecting against oxidative stress and inflammation. It also plays a role in the immune response and helps maintain a healthy gut environment. Brazil nuts, seafood, organ meats, and whole grains are sources of selenium. [17]

Potassium. This mineral is essential for proper muscle function, including the smooth muscles of the digestive tract. It helps regulate fluid balance, aids in nerve transmission, and supports overall gut health. Good sources of potassium include bananas, avocados, spinach, sweet potatoes, and white beans. [18]

Calcium. Known primarily for its role in bone health, calcium is also important for gut health. It helps regulate muscle contractions in the digestive tract and supports the proper function of enzymes involved in digestion. Leafy greens, such as kale and collard green, fortified plant-based milk, and sesame seeds are all excellent sources of calcium.[19]

Vitamin K. This vitamin plays a critical role in blood clotting, but it also has benefits for gut health. Vitamin K helps maintain the integrity of the gut lining and supports the production of certain bacteria that contribute to a healthy gut microbiome. Leafy green vegetables, such as kale, spinach, and broccoli, are rich sources of vitamin K. [20]

By prioritizing these essential minerals and vitamins in your diet, you can provide your gut with the necessary nutrients for optimal health and function. Choose a variety of nutrient-dense foods to ensure you're getting a wide range of vitamins and minerals to support your gut and overall well-being.

Sprouts

One category of highly nutritious foods that deserves special attention is sprouts. Sprouts are young plants that have just germinated from seeds, and they are packed with essential vitamins, minerals, enzymes, and antioxidants. [21]. Some of the best sprouts to include in your diet for gut health are:

Broccoli Sprouts. These tiny sprouts are rich in sulforaphane, a compound known for its anti-inflammatory and anticancer properties.

Alfalfa Sprouts. Loaded with vitamins A, C, and K, as well as minerals like calcium and potassium, alfalfa sprouts provide a nutritional boost to your salads and sandwiches.

Radish Sprouts. These spicy sprouts are high in vitamin C and contain compounds that support liver detoxification and digestion.

Sunflower Sprouts. With their nutty flavor, sunflower sprouts are a great source of protein, fiber, and essential nutrients like vitamin E and selenium.

Mung Bean Sprouts. These crunchy sprouts are a good source of vitamin C and contain enzymes that aid in digestion.

Superfood Powders

In addition to sprouts, certain "superfoods" in powdered form can be valuable additions to your diet. These powders are derived from nutrient-dense foods and offer concentrated amounts of essential nutrients. [22] Some notable superfood powders for gut health include:

Maca powder. Known for its adaptogenic properties, maca powder helps balance hormones and supports overall well-being.

Chlorella powder. This freshwater algae is rich in chlorophyll, which aids in detoxification and supports gut health.

Spirulina powder. Another type of algae, spirulina is packed with protein, essential amino acids, and various vitamins and minerals. It provides antioxidant and anti-inflammatory benefits.

Moringa powder. Derived from the leaves of the moringa tree, this powder is a nutrient powerhouse containing vitamins, minerals, antioxidants, and anti-inflammatory compounds.

Sea Kelp powder. Sea kelp is a type of seaweed that is high in iodine, which is important for thyroid function. It also contains other minerals and antioxidants that contribute to gut health.

Incorporating these nutrient-dense foods into your diet can provide a wealth of essential vitamins, minerals, and antioxidants to support your gut health. Please note that while this overview provides an introduction to the role of vitamins and minerals in gut health, it is always beneficial to consult with a healthcare professional or registered dietitian for personalized guidance and to address specific nutritional needs.

Proteins

Protein is an essential nutrient that plays a crucial role in supporting gut health. It is involved in various aspects of gut tissue repair, maintenance, and overall function. [23]

Protein is the building block of tissues, including the cells that line the gut. It plays a vital role in repairing damaged gut tissues and maintaining the integrity of the gut barrier. Adequate protein intake supports the growth and regeneration of gut cells, ensuring a healthy and functional digestive system. Protein aids in the synthesis of enzymes and hormones involved in digestion and nutrient absorption.

Best Sources of Protein

To support gut health, it is important to include high-quality protein sources in your diet. Opt for lean sources of protein that are rich in essential amino acids.

Here are some excellent options:

Lean meats

Fish and seafood

Legumes

Eggs

Dairy products

Plant-based protein

Lean meats. Choose lean cuts of poultry, such as skinless chicken breast and turkey. These meats provide high-quality protein along with essential vitamins and minerals.

Fish and seafood. Fatty fish like salmon, tuna, and sardines are not only excellent sources of protein but also rich in omega-3 fatty acids, which have anti-inflammatory properties as described earlier. Incorporating fish into your diet can benefit both your gut and overall health.

Legumes. Beans, lentils, and chickpeas are plant-based sources of protein that also offer dietary fiber, promoting a healthy gut microbiome. They are versatile and can be included in various dishes, such as soups, salads, and stews.

Eggs. Eggs are a complete protein source, meaning they contain all the essential amino acids your body needs. They are also rich in nutrients like choline and vitamin B12, which support brain and nervous system health.

Dairy products. Yogurt, Kefir, and cheeses are not only excellent sources of protein but also provide essential nutrients and probiotics.

Plant-based protein. For those following a vegetarian or vegan diet, plant-based protein sources like tofu, tempeh, quinoa, and edamame can provide the necessary protein. These options are also often rich in fiber and other beneficial nutrients.

Protein Powders

Protein powders offer a convenient and versatile way to supplement your protein intake. They can be beneficial for individuals with increased protein needs, athletes, or those who may have difficulty meeting their protein requirements through whole food sources alone. These are some of the benefits of protein powder and some popular types and sources.

Convenience. Protein powder is easy to incorporate into your daily routine. Simply mix it with water, milk, or your favorite beverage, or blend it into smoothies, shakes, or recipes. It provides a quick and portable source of high-quality protein, making it ideal for busy people.

Muscle recovery and growth. Protein powders are rich in essential amino acids, which are crucial for muscle repair and growth. Consuming protein powder after exercise can help replenish amino acid stores, support muscle recovery, and promote the development of lean muscle mass.

Weight Management. Protein is known for its ability to promote feelings of fullness and satiety, which can help curb appetite and support weight management goals. Incorporating protein powder into your meals or snacks can help increase protein content and aid in controlling cravings and overeating.

Diverse options. Protein powders come in many types to suit a variety of dietary preferences and needs.

Here are some popular options:

Whey protein. Derived from milk, whey protein is a complete protein source that contains all essential amino acids. It is quickly absorbed by the body and is used to support muscle recovery and growth.

Plant-based protein. Plant-based protein powders, such as pea, rice, hemp, or soy protein, offer options for individuals following vegetarian, vegan, or lactose-free diets. They provide a complete or complementary profile of amino acids and can be digested easily.

Collagen protein. Collagen protein powder is derived from animal sources, primarily bovine or marine collagen. It is rich in amino acids that support joint health, skin elasticity, and connective tissue maintenance.

Multi-source blends. Protein powders that combine different protein sources, such as whey, casein, and plant-based proteins, offer a balanced amino acid profile and provide a broader range of benefits.

Remember to choose high-quality protein powders from reputable brands that undergo third-party testing to ensure purity and safety. Read labels carefully to check for additional ingredients and be mindful of potential allergens or sensitivities.

It's important to note that while protein powders can be a convenient addition to your diet, they should not replace whole food sources of protein. Aim to get most of your protein from a well-rounded diet that includes lean meats, fish, legumes, fermented dairy products, eggs, and plant-based protein sources.

As with any dietary supplement, it is recommended to consult with a healthcare professional or registered dietitian before incorporating protein powder into your routine, especially if you have any underlying health conditions or specific dietary considerations.

Warning about dairy products

It is important to note that while dairy products can be a source of protein and nutrients like calcium and vitamin D, they may not be suitable for everyone's gut health. For many individuals, dairy products can contribute to gut-related issues and cause discomfort. [24]. The lactose and proteins present in dairy can be challenging to digest for some, leading to symptoms such as bloating, gas, and digestive disturbances.

If you find that dairy products do not agree with your gut, it may be beneficial to explore alternative sources of protein and nutrients. Fortunately, there are plenty of plant-based options available (plant-based milks, for example) that can provide similar benefits without the potential drawbacks. These alternatives can provide the necessary nutrients while being more gut-friendly for those who are sensitive to dairy.

It's essential to listen to your body and make choices that promote your well-being. Remember, the goal is to nourish and support your gut health through choices that work best for you. By being mindful of your body's responses and exploring suitable alternatives, you can find a balance that promotes both gut health and overall well-being.

Warning about animal protein sources

In this book, we are mindful of the potential impact of certain foods on gut health. As someone who has personally experienced the challenges of gut-related health issues, including leaky gut syndrome and autoimmune disease, I understand how important it is to make the right dietary choices that support healing and overall well-being.

One significant change I made on my health journey was eliminating red meat. After being diagnosed with leaky gut syndrome and an autoimmune disease in my 40s, I embarked on a mission to restore and nourish my gut health. Through extensive research and personal experimentation, I discovered that eliminating red meat from my diet played a crucial role in managing my symptoms and promoting gut healing.

Red meat has been associated with increased inflammation and potential disruption to the delicate balance of the gut microbiome, which can further exacerbate gut-related issues. [25] By transitioning to a predominantly plant-based diet and exploring vegetarian sources of protein, I found I could still meet my nutritional needs while supporting my gut health.

While this book primarily focuses on vegetarian sources of protein, with some recipes containing animal sources, it is important to recognize that dietary choices are individual. We each have unique needs and preferences, and it is essential to listen to our bodies and make choices that align with our well-being. For those who choose to incorporate animal-based protein sources, it's important to focus on mindful and balanced consumption.

By sharing my journey and the knowledge I have gained along the way, I hope to inspire and empower you to make choices that nourish your gut and support your overall health. Together, we will explore a diverse array of protein sources, discover delicious and satisfying recipes, and find a balance that resonates with your body and well-being.

Hormone Balancers

Hormonal balance plays a crucial role in managing menopause symptoms and promoting overall well-being during this transformative stage of life. The fluctuations in hormones that occur during menopause can give rise to various uncomfortable symptoms, including hot flashes, mood swings, sleep disturbances, and weight changes.

Understanding the role of hormone balancers in managing menopause symptoms is essential for navigating this phase of life with grace and vitality. Female hormone balancers help regulate hormonal fluctuations, promote harmony within the endocrine system, and support overall hormonal balance. By incorporating these hormone-balancing foods into our diet, we can support our body's natural processes and help mitigate the intensity and frequency of menopause symptoms, leading to a more comfortable and fulfilling life.

As someone who has personally experienced the challenges of menopause, I can attest to the power of hormone-balancing foods in managing these symptoms. After experiencing disruptive symptoms such as hot flashes, mood swings, and fatigue, I sought natural approaches to find relief and discovered the remarkable impact that certain foods can have on hormonal balance and ment.

Sources of Hormone Balancing Foods

Including hormone-balancing foods in our diet can provide substantial support during the menopause transition. These foods contain essential nutrients, phytochemicals, and bioactive compounds that help regulate hormone production and promote overall hormonal well-being. [26].

Here are some examples of hormone-balancing foods you can incorporate into your meals:

Flaxseeds

Non-GMO Organic Soy Products

Cruciferous Vegetables

Fatty fish

Nuts and Seeds

Herbal Teas: red clover, dong quai, and chamomile

Pomegranate

Foods High in Magnesium: leafy greens, almonds, pumpkin seeds, and legumes

Quinoa

Yams

Cherries

Lean Protein: chicken breast, turkey, and fish

..a Virgin Olive Oil

Avocados

Chia Seeds

Cinnamon

Ginger

Turmeric

Mushrooms: Nature's Healing Miracle Workers

Mushrooms have long been known as a treasure trove of nutritional and medicinal benefits. These remarkable fungi come in various shapes, sizes, and flavors, each offering its unique array of health properties. They are high in vitamins, minerals, protein, and essential amino acids. They act as natural antibiotics, reduce the risk of cancer and developing Alzheimer's disease, and help reduce high blood pressure. [27]

Incorporating mushrooms into your diet can bring a delightful twist to your meals while providing many benefits for your overall well-being, gut health, and menopause symptoms. Let's explore some of the fascinating mushrooms and their extraordinary qualities.

White button mushrooms. These mild-flavored mushrooms are packed with nutrients like vitamins B2, B3, and B5, as well as selenium, copper, and potassium. They are also known for their immune-boosting properties due to the presence of beta-glucans, which can enhance the activity of immune cells.

Cremini mushrooms. Similar in appearance to white button mushrooms, cremini mushrooms offer a deeper, earthier flavor. They contain a range of B vitamins, as well as minerals like selenium and copper. Cremini mushrooms are also an excellent source of ergothioneine, a powerful antioxidant that may help protect against oxidative stress.

Porcini mushrooms. Prized for their rich, nutty flavor, porcini mushrooms are not only delicious but also provide a good dose of vitamins, minerals, and antioxidants. They are high in potassium, which is essential for maintaining healthy blood pressure and heart function.

Portobello mushrooms. Portobello mushrooms are mature cremini mushrooms that have developed a meatier texture and deeper flavor. These mushrooms are a wonderful source of fiber, selenium, and B vitamins. They are also known for their high antioxidant content, which helps combat oxidative damage in the body.

Chanterelle mushrooms. Culinary enthusiasts prize these mushrooms for their golden color and delicate flavor. They are a good source of vitamins C and D, which play important roles in immune function and bone health. Chanterelle mushrooms also contain antioxidants that may help protect against inflammation.

Oyster mushrooms. Oyster mushrooms have a delicate, seafood-like taste and a tender texture. They are low in calories and rich in nutrients like fiber, vitamin D, and iron. Oyster mushrooms also contain lovastatin, a compound that has been shown to help regulate cholesterol levels.

Reishi mushrooms. Known as the “Queen of Mushrooms,” Reishi mushrooms have been revered for their immune-boosting properties. They contain bioactive compounds that can help regulate immune function, reduce inflammation, and support overall gut health. Incorporating Reishi mushrooms into your diet may contribute to managing menopause symptoms by promoting a balanced immune response.

Shiitake mushrooms. Shiitake mushrooms contain a powerful compound, a polysaccharide called lentinan, known for its immune-enhancing properties. They are a rich source of beta-glucans, which can support gut health by nourishing beneficial gut bacteria and promoting a healthy gut environment.

Lion's Mane mushrooms. Lion's Mane mushrooms have gained popularity for their potential cognitive benefits. These mushrooms contain compounds that may support brain health, memory, and focus. They can reduce the risk of age-related cognitive decline. Incorporating Lion's Mane mushrooms into your diet during menopause may provide additional support for cognitive well-being.

Cordyceps mushrooms. These mushrooms have been traditionally used in herbal medicine to enhance vitality and energy. They have adaptogenic properties, meaning they can help the body adapt to stress and promote overall resilience. Cordyceps mushrooms may support energy levels and physical performance during menopause, helping you maintain an active and vibrant lifestyle.

Maitake mushrooms. Maitake mushrooms, also known as "Hen of the Woods," offer a range of health-promoting compounds. Like Shiitake, they contain beta-glucans. Maitake mushrooms have been studied for their potential to regulate blood sugar levels, which may be beneficial for managing hormonal imbalances associated with menopause.

Including a variety of mushrooms in your diet can be a flavorful and beneficial choice. Whether you sauté them, add them to soups and stews, or enjoy them as a meat substitute, mushrooms provide a wealth of nutrients, including vitamins, minerals, fiber, and antioxidants. They can contribute to gut health by supporting a diverse gut microbiome and promoting a healthy balance of gut bacteria.

As you navigate the menopause journey, incorporating mushrooms into your meals can provide you with an extra dose of nature's healing power. Embrace the magic of mushrooms and savor their unique flavors and health properties as you nourish your body.

Mushroom "Coffee"

In recent years, mushroom coffee has emerged as a trendy and innovative way to enjoy the benefits of mushrooms in your daily cup of java. Mushroom coffee is a unique blend of ground coffee beans and medicinal mushrooms. This combination not only offers a rich and flavorful coffee experience but also provides an added dose of mushroom goodness.

Mushroom coffee has gained popularity because of its potential to enhance focus and mental clarity. The combination of caffeine from the coffee beans and the natural compounds found in mushrooms creates a synergistic effect that can promote cognitive function and support a balanced mood.

You can buy mushroom "coffee" powder blends in any health food store or in many grocery stores. They often contain the following ingredients: Lion's Mane, Chaga, Cordyceps, Reishi, Carob, Maca powder, MCT oil, Cocoa, Cinnamon, Rooibos, and Himalayan Salt.

For me, discovering mushroom coffee was an exciting revelation in my quest for natural ways to manage menopause symptoms and enhance my overall health. As a coffee lover, I was thrilled to find a beverage that also offered additional benefits through medicinal mushrooms. Incorporating mushroom coffee into my daily routine has become a delightful and invigorating experience that has contributed to my well-being during the menopause journey.

By embracing mushroom coffee, you can enjoy the comforting and energizing effects of your favorite beverage while reaping the potential benefits of medicinal mushrooms. It's a delicious way to incorporate the magic of mushrooms into your daily routine.

Nature's Little Secrets: Herbs for Better Health

Herbs have long been revered for their potent healing properties and their ability to enhance the flavor and nutritional value of our meals. These incredible plants are packed with essential vitamins, minerals, and antioxidants that contribute to overall health. Incorporating herbs into our diet can not only add depth and complexity to our dishes but also provide a range of health benefits. [28]

Herbs are known for their anti-inflammatory, antimicrobial, and antioxidant properties, making them valuable allies in supporting immune function, reducing inflammation, and protecting against chronic diseases. Additionally, many herbs have been used traditionally to aid digestion, promote healthy circulation, and balance hormones.

Here are some of the most popular herbs and their unique properties:

Basil. Known for its anti-inflammatory properties and rich in antioxidants, basil adds a burst of freshness and flavor to your dishes.

Rosemary. With its distinctive aroma and taste, rosemary is not only a flavorful addition but also contains compounds that may improve digestion and enhance cognitive function.

Thyme. This herb is a powerhouse of antioxidants and has antimicrobial properties that support immune health and combat infections.

Oregano. Known for its antibacterial and antifungal properties, oregano is a versatile herb that adds a savory touch to your meals.

Mint. Refreshing and soothing mint is commonly used to aid digestion and alleviate symptoms of indigestion.

Cilantro (Coriander). This herb is packed with vitamins and minerals and helps detoxify the body and reduce inflammation.

Dill. Vitamins and minerals in dill include vitamin D, riboflavin, iron, and calcium. They support bone health, the immune function, and protect the cells from free radical damage.

The Gut Offenders

When it comes to maintaining a healthy gut and managing menopause symptoms, it is crucial to be aware of the foods that can undermine our efforts and compromise gut health. These are the gut offenders—the foods that have been shown to have detrimental effects on the gut microbiome and may worsen menopausal symptoms. Understanding these culprits will empower us to make informed dietary choices that promote gut health and overall well-being during perimenopause and menopause.

Processed foods. Processed foods, such as packaged snacks, frozen meals, and fast food items, are often high in unhealthy additives, preservatives, and artificial ingredients. These components can disrupt the delicate balance of the gut microbiota and contribute to gut dysbiosis and inflammation. It is important to avoid processed foods and instead choose whole, unprocessed alternatives that are rich in nutrients and support a healthy gut.

High-sugar foods. Excessive consumption of high-sugar foods, including sugary drinks, candies, pastries, and sweetened desserts, has been associated with various health issues, including gut dysbiosis, inflammation, and impaired gut barrier function. Menopausal women may be particularly susceptible to the negative effects of high-sugar foods on gut health. Choosing naturally sweet options like fruits and honey and minimizing added sugars in the diet can help maintain a healthy gut environment.

Certain fats and oils. Some fats and oils are detrimental to gut health. Trans fats and hydrogenated oils, palm oil, often found in fried foods, processed snacks, and margarine, have been shown to promote inflammation and disrupt the gut microbiota. Excessive intake of saturated fats, commonly found in fatty meats and full-fat dairy products, may negatively impact gut health and increase the risk of gut-related disorders. Opting for healthier fat sources like avocado oil, coconut oil, and olive oil can support a more favorable gut environment.

By being mindful of these gut offenders and making conscious choices to limit or avoid them, we can create an environment in our gut that supports optimal health and menopause management. Prioritizing a diet rich in whole, unprocessed foods and minimizing the consumption of processed foods, high-sugar foods, and unhealthy fats can help maintain a healthy gut microbiome and reduce inflammation.

Intermittent Fasting and Gut-Healthy Recipes

In my first book, I introduced the "Skip a Meal" habit of Intermittent Fasting, a powerful approach that can become a game changer for your gut health journey. While the recipes in this book follow a structure of three nourishing meals a day, I understand our lifestyles vary. The beauty of intermittent fasting lies in its flexibility, and this habit can seamlessly merge with the recipes, enhancing their benefits.

Skipping Breakfast

If you relish the idea of dinner as a social or family meal, this popular method of intermittent fasting may be best for you. Start your day with a hydrating herbal tea or a glass of water to awaken your digestive system. Continue your fasting window until lunchtime by drinking coffee, tea, and plenty of water. Enjoy your nutrient-packed smoothie for lunch to provide your body with the essential nutrients to kick-start your feeding window. This approach ensures that your smoothie remains the cornerstone of your daily routine while aligning with the principles of intermittent fasting.

Sometimes you might find it more suitable to enjoy your big salad for lunch. In this case, feel free to alternate smoothies and salads on different days depending on your lifestyle, work, and family circumstances, to keep your meals interesting and satisfying.

Skipping Dinner

If you cannot imagine starting your day without a nourishing breakfast, skipping dinner might be the perfect strategy for you. It recognizes that some people thrive with a robust morning routine and require substantial energy to kick-start their day. By skipping dinner instead of breakfast, you're ensuring that your body receives the essential nutrients it needs for the day ahead.

When you aim for weight loss, dinner fasting can offer an advantage. From my experience, fasting in the evening can support weight management better by giving your body more time to burn calories. It also helps some women reduce the likelihood of overeating or snacking before bedtime.

Balancing soups and salads for lunch as the last meal of the day can be a smart approach to optimizing your nutrient intake and promoting gut health. By alternating between these two options, you can provide your body with a range of nutrients while enjoying a variety of flavors, textures, and nutrients and supporting optimal digestion.

You can experiment with different schedules and find the rhythm that resonates with your body and lifestyle. With all fasting methods, it's essential to listen to your body and assess how each approach affects your energy levels and overall health. Talking to your doctor is always a good idea to make any important decision about your health. By discovering what resonates with you, you can confidently tailor your intermittent fasting strategy to optimize your unique needs.

Intermittent fasting can be seamlessly aligned with the nourishing recipes in this book. Whether you're a morning person, a lunchtime enthusiast, or prefer evening rituals, there's a fasting approach that can complement your lifestyle. The key is to honor your body's needs and cultivate habits that support your well-being on a path to holistic vitality.

What's Ahead

This chapter has taken us on a journey through the world of food groups that fuel our gut and promote a healthy digestive system. We have explored the incredible benefits of fiber-rich foods in supporting gut health and regulating digestion. We have explored the importance of prebiotics and their ability to nourish the beneficial bacteria in our gut. We unveiled the role of probiotics and fermented foods in maintaining a balanced gut microbiome. We have witnessed how significant omega-3 fatty acids are in promoting gut health and their potential benefits for cardiovascular and cognitive well-being. And we have learned about the anti-inflammatory, antioxidant, and hormonal balancing properties of certain foods.

As I embarked on my journey towards a healthier gut, I became fascinated by the abundance of healthy, whole foods and their incredible potential to enhance well-being. I experimented with incorporating these foods into my cooking, creating delicious and nourishing meals that not only satisfied my taste buds but also provided a myriad of health benefits. From fiber-rich greens to antioxidant-packed berries, each ingredient became a vital part of my meals, helping me nourish my gut and revitalize my entire body. These foods are my superheroes, armed with an arsenal of nutrients and bioactive compounds that work wonders.

As we turn the page to the next chapter, get ready to embark on a culinary adventure. We're diving into the world of smoothies, salads, and soups designed to nourish our bodies and minds. We'll explore the world of nutrient-packed smoothies that will kick-start our mornings with a burst of energy and vitality. We'll delve into the realm of salads, where we'll create vibrant and satisfying meals that support our gut health. And last but not least, we'll savor the comforting hug of wholesome and nourishing soups.

So, girlfriend, gather your blenders, bowls, and pots because we're about to celebrate the power of food to heal, rejuvenate, and support our gut health. Get ready to discover a world of flavors, textures, and endless possibilities!

3

Morning Kickstart: Smoothie Recipes

When it comes to starting our day on a nourishing note, there's something truly magical about the power of a smoothie. This vibrant concoction, packed with a medley of wholesome ingredients, has the potential to unlock a world of ageless vitality and rejuvenation.

It was during my quest for improved health that I discovered the transformative power of smoothies. As I was managing menopause and autoimmune symptoms, improving gut health, and pursuing sustainable weight loss, I bought a blender. And I found a wealth of nutrients in blended drinks.

Smoothies quickly became an integral part of my daily routine, providing me with a convenient and delicious way to nourish my body. I experimented with an array of flavors, combining nutrient-rich fruits, leafy greens, spices, and other gut-friendly ingredients. Each sip was like a burst of vitality, infusing my body with the goodness it craved.

Not only did smoothies become a vital tool in managing my menopause symptoms, but they also played a crucial role in healing my leaky gut. I witnessed the remarkable impact they had on my digestion, energy levels, and overall well-being. They became a cornerstone of my journey toward restored health, helping me find balance and harmony in my body.

But what makes smoothies so special? Let's discover the reasons behind their popularity.

Why Smoothies?

Smoothies are not just delicious. They also offer remarkable benefits for our gut health and overall health. Blending ingredients into a smooth, drinkable consistency can enhance digestion by breaking down fibers and releasing the nutrients hidden within. This process makes it easier for our bodies to absorb these essential nutrients, ensuring that we reap the full benefits of the ingredients. By incorporating fiber-rich fruits, vegetables, and other gut-healthy ingredients into our smoothies, we provide our digestive system with the support it needs to function optimally.

Smoothies offer a convenient and versatile way to nourish our bodies. Whether you prefer a quick grab-and-go option for busy mornings or a leisurely moment to savor your favorite blend, smoothies can suit any lifestyle. With unlimited combinations of flavors, textures, and nutritional profiles, you can customize them to cater to your taste and health goals. From vibrant green creations to luscious berry and citrus blends, the possibilities are endless.

The role of smoothies in maintaining gut function

Staying hydrated is essential for overall health, including our gut health. Smoothies are an excellent source of hydration, especially when you incorporate hydrating ingredients such as juicy fruits and coconut water. These liquid components provide a refreshing boost of hydration, ensuring that our bodies stay nourished and our digestive system functions well. [29]

Smoothies also contribute to maintaining a healthy gut environment. By including gut-friendly ingredients such as prebiotics and probiotics, we nourish beneficial bacteria in our digestive system and support a diverse and thriving gut microbiome. This promotes better digestion, improved nutrient absorption, and a strengthened immune system. Smoothies are a convenient and enjoyable way to incorporate these gut-nourishing ingredients into our daily routine.

How to Prepare Smoothies: Step-by-Step Guide

Preparing a delicious and nutritious smoothie is a breeze when you follow these simple steps.

1. Wash and prepare. Start by washing all the fruits, vegetables, and leafy greens you plan to use. Remove any hard stems, pits, or inedible parts. This ensures your ingredients are ready to be blended.

2. Chop and slice. Depending on the power of your blender, it may be beneficial to chop or slice larger ingredients into smaller pieces. This helps facilitate blending and ensures a smooth consistency in your finished smoothie.

3. Add Liquid Base. Pour your preferred liquid into the blender first. The amount of liquid may vary depending on the desired thickness of your smoothie. Start with about 1 cup and adjust as needed.

4. Add greens and fresh fruits and vegetables. Next, add your leafy greens, such as spinach, kale, etc. Then, add all other fruits and vegetables like apples, mango, cucumber, avocado, celery, carrots, etc.

5. Add frozen fruits and veggies. If you use any frozen ingredients, now is the time to add them.

6. Add protein and other powders and superfoods. This can include spirulina, maca powder, moringa powder, any protein powder, chia seeds, flaxseeds, soaked seeds and nuts, etc.

7. Add ice. Ice cubes go last if you want to add them. Ice helps to pull all ingredients together to reach a smooth consistency. However, if you use frozen fruit or veggies, you may not need it.

8. Blend until smooth. Secure the lid of your blender and blend at high speed until all the ingredients are well combined, and the smoothie has a creamy texture. This takes about 1-2 minutes, but you can adjust the blending time based on your preference for texture.

9. Taste and adjust. Give your smoothie a quick taste and adjust the flavor if needed. You can also add more ice for better smoothness.

10. Count your chews. And last but not least, remember your healthy gut habit number 3 when enjoying your delicious creation. Although smoothies are liquid, it's important to "chew" them by swishing them in your mouth before swallowing. This simple act stimulates the production of saliva, which begins breaking down the food and preparing it for digestion. Chewing also signals the stomach to produce digestive juices, ensuring optimal nutrient absorption. So, take a moment to savor each sip, allowing your taste buds and digestive system to fully appreciate the nourishing goodness of your smoothie. This reminder will help you make the most out of your experience and support the optimal digestion and absorption of nutrients. Enjoy your smoothies mindfully!

With these simple steps, you can prepare a variety of smoothies to suit your taste preferences and nutritional needs. Even if you follow the recipes in this book, you can still get creative with your ingredient combinations, so experiment with different ingredients, flavors, and textures. Here are a few tips on how you can do that.

Tips to Customize Smoothie Recipes

Creating your own personalized smoothie is an exciting adventure that allows you to cater to your unique taste preferences, dietary needs, and the availability of seasonal ingredients.

1. Flavorful Additions. Experiment with different flavor enhancers such as spices (cinnamon, nutmeg, ginger, allspice, etc.), natural extracts (vanilla, almond), or superfood powders (maca, spirulina, carob, cocoa) to elevate the taste of your smoothie.

2. Sweetness Level. Adjust the sweetness of your smoothie by adding natural sweeteners like honey, maple syrup, dates, monk fruit, or stevia. If you prefer a less sweet smoothie, rely on the natural sweetness of the fruits. Remember, fruit is very high in sugar, especially dried fruit.

3. Texture and Creaminess: Customize the texture of your smoothie by adding ice cubes for a frosty blend or using frozen fruits to create a thicker consistency. For extra creaminess, incorporate ingredients like avocado, yogurt, banana, organic tofu, nut and seed butter.

4. Nutrient Boosters: Tailor your smoothie to your specific dietary needs by adding nutrient boosters like ground flaxseeds, flaxseed oil, MCT oil, chia seeds, hemp hearts, or protein powders to enhance the nutritional content.

5. Seasonal Variations: Embrace the flavors of each season by incorporating seasonal fruits and vegetables into your smoothies. This not only ensures freshness but also adds variety and supports local and sustainable food choices.

With the knowledge of the benefits and versatility of smoothies, it's time to dive into the recipes.

Note: The preparation time for all smoothies is approximately 10 min. The quantities provided are for 2 servings. Adjust the ingredient amounts based on your desired consistency, taste, and appetite.

Green Powerhouses

1. Green Goddess Breakfast

- 1 cup coconut water or filtered water
- 1 cup baby spinach
- 1 cup kale leaves
- 1/2 frozen banana
- 1/2 cucumber, peeled and sliced
- 2 broccoli florets
- 1/2 avocado
- 1 tablespoon chia seeds
- a handful of fresh mint leaves
- a few ice cubes

2. Refreshing Green Citrus

- 1 cup green tea, chilled
- 1 cup baby spinach
- 1 cup mustard greens

- 1 small orange, segmented
- 1/2 grapefruit, segmented
- 1 tablespoon flaxseeds
- a few sprigs of fresh cilantro
- a few ice cubes

3. Minty Matcha Blast

- 1 cup unsweetened almond milk
- 2 cups Swiss chard leaves
- 1 banana
- 1 teaspoon Matcha green tea powder
- 1 tablespoon almond butter
- 1/2 teaspoon cinnamon
- a few fresh mint leaves
- a few ice cubes

4. Green Detox Smoothie

- 1 cup coconut water or filtered water
- 1/2 cup dandelion greens
- 1/2 cup mustard greens

- 1/2 cup collard greens
- 1/2 cup chopped celery
- 1/2 frozen banana
- 1/4 cucumber, peeled and sliced
- 1/2 lemon, juiced
- 1-inch piece of ginger, chopped
- 1 tablespoon chia seeds
- a few ice cubes

5. Super Green Energy Boost

- 1 cup unsweetened almond milk
- 1 cup spinach
- 1/2 cup kale
- 1/2 avocado
- 1/2 cup frozen green grapes
- 1 frozen banana chunks
- 1 tablespoon chia seeds
- 1 teaspoon spirulina powder
- a drizzle of honey or maple syrup

6. Lady Moringa

- 1 cup coconut water or filtered water
- 1 cup baby spinach
- 2 broccoli florets
- 1/2 cucumber, peeled and sliced
- 1/2 green apple, cored and chopped
- 1 tablespoon Moringa powder
- 1 tablespoon hemp seeds
- a handful of fresh mint leaves
- a few ice cubes

Prebiotic Paradise

7. Prebiotic Berry Bliss

- 1 cup unsweetened almond milk
- 1 cup mixed berries
- 1 banana
- 1 cup dandelion greens
- 1/2 cup rolled oats
- 1 tablespoon chia seeds

- 1 tablespoon ground flaxseeds
- a few ice cubes

8. Creamy Banana-Blueberry Blend

- 1 cup unsweetened oat milk
- 1 banana
- 1/2 cup blueberries
- 1/2 cup cooked quinoa
- 1 tablespoon almond butter
- 1 tablespoon ground flaxseeds
- a sprinkle of cinnamon
- a few ice cubes

9. Apple - Walnut Prebiotic Boost

- 1 cup unsweetened almond milk
- 1 green apple, cored and chopped
- 1/2 cup chopped celery
- 1/4 cup walnuts, soaked overnight
- 1 tablespoon ground flaxseeds
- 1 tablespoon maple syrup

- a pinch of cinnamon
- a few ice cubes

10. Purple Paradise

- 1 cup unsweetened almond milk
- 1/2 cup cooked purple sweet potatoes
- 1/2 cup pitted frozen cherries
- 1/2 cup rolled oats
- 1/2 cup shredded red cabbage
- 1 tablespoon almond butter
- a few ice cubes

11. Orange Sunset

- 1 cup coconut milk
- 1 cup chopped carrots
- 1/2 cup cooked yam chunks
- 1/2 cup papaya chunks
- 1 banana
- 1 small orange, segmented
- 1/2 teaspoon turmeric

- a few ice cubes

12. Red Velvet

- 1 cup of coconut water or filtered water
- 1 cup mixed fresh or frozen pitted cherries and/or strawberries
- 1/2 cup fresh watermelon chunks
- 2 chopped dates
- 1/4 cup chopped beets
- 1 banana
- a few ice cubes

Hormonal Harmony

13. Berry-Beet Hormone Harmony

- 1/2 cup unsweetened almond milk
- 1/2 cup Greek yogurt (or non-dairy yogurt)
- 1/2 cup pomegranate juice
- 1 cup frozen mixed berries (strawberries, raspberries, blueberries)
- 1/2 cup cranberries
- 1 small beet, peeled and diced

- 1 tablespoon flaxseeds
- a few ice cubes

14. Hemp Goddess Balancer

- 1/2 cup coconut water
- 1/2 cup unsweetened almond milk
- 1 cup spinach
- 2 broccoli florets
- 1/2 ripe avocado
- 1/2 frozen banana chunks
- 1 tablespoon hemp hearts
- 1 tablespoon almond butter
- 1 tablespoon pumpkin seeds
- a few ice cubes

15. Maca-Mango Magic

- 1 cup coconut milk
- 1 cup frozen mango chunks
- 1 tablespoon maca powder
- 1/2 cup cooked quinoa

- 1 tablespoon chia seeds
- 1/2 teaspoon ground cinnamon
- a few ice cubes

16. Golden Turmeric Bliss

- 1 cup unsweetened almond milk
- 1 frozen banana chunks
- 1/2 cup cooked yam
- 1/2 teaspoon ground turmeric
- a pinch of black pepper
- 1 teaspoon chopped ginger
- 1 tablespoon flaxseeds
- 1 tablespoon honey or maple syrup
- a few ice cubes

17. Silky Mocha Elixir

- 1 cup unsweetened almond milk
- 1/2 cup silken tofu, drained
- 1 tablespoon unsweetened cocoa powder
- 1 banana

- 1 tablespoon honey
- a sprinkle of ground cinnamon
- a few ice cubes

Gut Soothing Elixirs

18. Pineapple Ginger Zinger

- 1 cup coconut water or filtered water
- 1 cup fresh pineapple chunks
- 1-inch piece of fresh ginger
- 1/2 cucumber, peeled and chopped
- 1 tablespoon fresh mint leaves
- 1 tablespoon flaxseed oil
- a squeeze of fresh lime juice
- a few ice cubes

19. Creamy Banana-Oat Soother

- 1 cup unsweetened almond milk
- 1/2 banana
- 1/3 cup papaya chunks
- 1/2 cup cooked oats

- 2 Brazil nuts, soaked overnight
- 1/3 cup cooked sweet potato
- 1 tablespoon almond butter
- 1/2 teaspoon ground cinnamon
- a few ice cubes

20. Cooling Cucumber-Mint Delight

- 1/2 cup coconut water or filtered water
- 1/2 cup Greek yogurt (or non-dairy yogurt)
- 1/2 cucumber, peeled and sliced
- 1/2 cup fresh spinach leaves
- 1/2 avocado
- 1/4 cup fresh mint leaves
- 1/2 teaspoon Matcha green tea powder
- a squeeze of fresh lemon juice
- a few ice cubes

21. Healing Aloe Vera Elixir

- 1 cup coconut water
- 1 cup kale

- 1/4 cup pure aloe vera gel
- 1/2 cup sliced cucumber
- 1 tablespoon fresh lemon juice
- 1 tablespoon hemp hearts
- 1 teaspoon honey or maple syrup
- a few fresh basil leaves
- a few ice cubes

22. Berry-Licious Gut Soother

- 1/2 cup unsweetened almond milk
- 1/2 cup Greek yogurt (or non-dairy yogurt)
- 1 cup frozen mixed berries
- 1/2 cup cooked or canned and drained chickpeas
- 1 tablespoon sunflower seeds, soaked
- 1 tablespoon ground flaxseeds
- a few ice cubes

23. Chocolate Matcha Delight

- 1 cup almond milk
- 1 frozen banana

- 1 tablespoon cocoa powder
- 1 teaspoon Matcha green tea powder
- 1 tablespoon almond butter
- 1/2 teaspoon cinnamon
- a sprinkle of cacao nibs, optional
- a few ice cubes

Protein-Packed Smoothies

24. Creamy Coconut-Berry Blast

- 1/2 cup coconut milk
- 1/2 cup Greek yogurt (or non-dairy yogurt)
- 1 cup mixed berries (strawberries, blueberries, raspberries)
- 1 scoop vanilla protein powder
- 1 tablespoon almond butter
- a few ice cubes

25. Chocolate-Banana Powerhouse

- 1 cup unsweetened almond milk
- 1 frozen banana chunks
- 1 scoop of chocolate protein powder

- 1 tablespoon chia seeds
- 1 tablespoon cocoa powder
- 1/2 cup baby spinach
- a few ice cubes

26. Tropical Island Protein Boost

- 1/2 cup coconut water or filtered water
- 1/3 cup pineapple chunks
- 1/3 cup mango chunks
- 1/3 cup papaya chunks
- 1 scoop vanilla protein powder
- 1 tablespoon flaxseeds
- a few ice cubes

27. Almond - Banana Protein Shake

- 1 cup unsweetened almond milk
- 1 frozen banana chunks
- 1 scoop peanut butter protein powder
- 1 tablespoon almond butter
- 1 tablespoon honey

- a sprinkle of cinnamon
- a few ice cubes

28. Green Power Protein Smoothie

- 1/2 cup Greek yogurt (or non-dairy yogurt)
- 1/2 cup almond milk
- 1/2 cup spinach leaves
- 1/2 cup dandelion greens
- 1 scoop vanilla protein powder
- 1 tablespoon seed butter
- a few ice cubes

Probiotic Powerhouses

29. Berry Kefir Blast

- 1/2 cup kefir
- 1/3 cup fresh or frozen mixed berries (strawberries, blueberries, raspberries)
- 1/3 cup frozen cranberries
- 1/3 cup frozen pitted cherries
- 1 frozen banana chunks

- 1 tablespoon chia seeds
- a drizzle of honey or maple syrup
- a few ice cubes

30. Mango Lassi Smoothie

- 1/2 cup Greek yogurt
- 1/2 cup coconut yogurt
- 1 cup mango chunks
- 1 tablespoon maca powder
- a sprinkle of cardamom powder
- a few ice cubes

31. Green Kombucha Elixir

- 1/2 cup lemon-lime kombucha (or any flavor of your choice)
- 1 cup spinach
- 1/2 cup cucumber, sliced
- 1/2 cup pineapple chunks
- 1 tablespoon lime juice
- 1 tablespoon lemon juice
- a few ice cubes

32. Strawberry Maca Smoothie

- 1/2 cup Greek yogurt
- 1/2 cup almond milk
- 2 cups fresh or frozen strawberries
- 1 tablespoon maca powder
- 1 teaspoon honey
- a few ice cubes

33. Creamy Coconut Kefir Delight

- 1/2 cup coconut yogurt
- 1/2 cup kefir
- 1 frozen banana chunks
- 1 tablespoon shredded coconut
- a sprinkle of cinnamon
- a few ice cubes

34. Blueberry Ginger Smoothie

- 1 cup ginger kombucha
- 1 cup fresh or frozen blueberries
- 1 cup watermelon chunks

- 1 frozen banana chunks
- 1 tablespoon honey
- 1 tablespoon lemon juice
- a few ice cubes

35. Chai Delight

- 1/2 cup Greek yogurt or coconut yogurt
- 1/2 cup black tea, chilled
- 1/2 cup silken tofu
- 1 frozen banana chunks
- 1 tablespoon honey
- 1 teaspoon chopped ginger
- 1/4 teaspoon cardamom
- 1/4 teaspoon cinnamon
- 1/4 teaspoon ground cloves
- a few ice cubes

Mushroom Magic

36. Mushroom Mocha

- 1 cup brewed coffee or decaf, chilled

- 1 cup almond milk
- 1 frozen banana chunks
- 1 tablespoon mushroom "coffee" blend
- 1 tablespoon unsweetened cocoa powder
- 1 tablespoon almond butter
- 2 dates, pitted and chopped
- a few ice cubes

37. Mushroom Matcha

- 1 cup green tea, chilled
- 1/2 cup coconut milk
- 1 frozen mango
- 1 tablespoon mushroom "coffee" blend
- 1 teaspoon Matcha green tea powder
- 1 tablespoon honey
- a few ice cubes

38. Golden Mushroom Elixir

- 1 cup unsweetened almond milk
- 1 frozen banana chunks

- 1 tablespoon mushroom “coffee” blend
- 1/2 teaspoon turmeric powder
- 1/2 teaspoon ginger powder
- 1 tablespoon honey or maple syrup
- a pinch of black pepper
- a few ice cubes

39. Reishi Cocoa Smoothie

- 1 cup unsweetened chocolate almond milk
- 1/2 cup Greek yogurt
- 1/2 avocado
- 1/2 frozen banana
- 1 tablespoon Reishi mushroom powder
- 1 tablespoon cocoa powder
- 1/2 frozen blueberries
- 1 teaspoon chia seeds
- a few ice cubes

With our smoothie creations for breakfast, we have nourished our bodies with these invigorating blends. Now it’s time to turn our attention to another culinary delight.

Join me for lunch in the next chapter as we explore a medley of vibrant salad recipes to keep you energized throughout the day.

4

Mid-Day Recharge: Salad Recipes

In my first book, "7 Healthy Gut Habits for Women over 40," I shared my love for "big salads" and how they have become a staple in my daily routine. It's interesting that growing up, salads were not an important part of my family's menu. It was only when I moved to Canada that I opened the delightful world of salads for myself. I later discovered that the term "big salad" came from an episode of Seinfeld where Elaine coined it after trying to order a big salad in a restaurant. You may remember that she was offered two small salads instead. Around that time, salads have become an important part of my culinary repertoire. First, it was because I just loved experimenting with a delightful array of flavors and textures and creating "eye candies" for my family. Later, they helped me on the journey toward optimal health, offering me the perfect opportunity to nourish and recharge during a busy day. All while delivering a powerhouse of essential nutrients to support my overall health and well-being.

Salads are more than just a side dish or a boring plate of greens. When done right, they can be a culinary masterpiece that excites all senses and leaves you feeling energized and satisfied. Over the years, I have mastered the art of combining vegetables, fruits, proteins, and dressings to make delicious and nutritious salads.

In this chapter, we will explore the art of salad making and dive into a collection of my favorite salad recipes. From gut-boosting greens to hormone-friendly combinations, anti-inflammatory bowls, and protein-packed creations, each recipe is crafted to provide a satisfying and nutrient-dense meal that will leave you feeling rejuvenated.

Whether you're a salad enthusiast or looking to incorporate more wholesome and delicious meals into your day, these recipes will inspire you to re-imagine the possibilities of a salad. Let's create vibrant and satisfying salads together, one delicious bite at a time.

The Art of Salad Making

Balance Various Food Elements for a Satisfying and Nutritious Salad

Creating a satisfying and nutritious salad requires a careful balance of various food elements. Here are the key components that make up a well-rounded salad:

Base greens. Start with fresh leafy greens like spinach, kale, arugula, fennel, or mixed salad greens. These greens provide essential vitamins, minerals, and fiber.

Vibrant vegetables. Add a variety of colorful vegetables such as tomatoes, cucumbers, bell peppers, carrots, or radishes. They provide an array of vitamins, and antioxidants, and add a crunchy touch.

Complex carbohydrates. Include roasted yams or sweet potatoes, millet, farro, quinoa, or brown rice, to provide sustained energy, prebiotics, and fiber.

Protein. Incorporate a source of protein to make your salad more filling and nourishing. Options include lean chicken, mushrooms, tofu, beans, salmon, or boiled eggs. More about it below.

Healthy fats. Don't forget to include healthy fats such as avocado, nuts, seeds, flaxseed oil, or extra virgin olive oil. These fats not only add richness and flavor but also aid in the absorption of fat-soluble vitamins.

Probiotics-rich foods. As you already know, probiotics are crucial for our gut health. We can enrich salads with probiotics by adding different fermented vegetables, yogurt, and cheeses.

Sprouts. Elevate the nutritional profile of your salad by including a handful of fresh sprouts. Simply rinse them gently, drain excess water, and scatter them atop your greens. These tender sprouts add a delightful crunch and an extra burst of freshness.

Flavorful additions. Enhance the taste and nutrition profile of your salad with fresh herbs, citrus zest, dried fruits, candied nuts, or crumbled cheeses. These additions elevate the flavor, add amazing health benefits, and bring a delightful twist to your salad.

Tips for Preparing Ahead and Storing Salads

Preparing salads ahead of time can save you valuable minutes during busy days. Here are some tips for prepping and storing salads to maintain their freshness and quality:

Wash and dry greens. Wash and spin-dry your greens before assembling the salad. Moisture can lead to wilting, so it's essential to remove excess water.

Separate wet and dry ingredients. Keep wet ingredients, such as tomatoes or dressings, separate from dry ingredients to prevent sogginess. Prepare and pack dressings separately in small containers to add right before serving.

Layering technique. Use a layering technique when packing salads to keep them fresh and crisp. Start with sturdier ingredients at the bottom and place delicate greens on top to prevent wilting.

Reliable containers. Invest in sturdy and airtight containers that will prevent leaks and keep your salad ingredients fresh. Glass and metal containers are the best, because plastic containers, even those BPA-Free, have been associated with various health problems.

Animal Protein Options for Gut-Healthy Salad Additions

While plant-based proteins are often emphasized for their gut health benefits, animal protein can also play a role in creating satisfying and nutrient-rich salads. If you choose to incorporate animal protein into your salads, it's important to opt for lean and gut-friendly options. Here are some animal protein options that can be a great addition to your gut-healthy salads:

Grilled chicken breast is a lean source of protein that adds a boost of flavor and texture to your salads. It's low in saturated fat and provides essential amino acids necessary for tissue repair and maintenance.

Salmon is an excellent source of omega-3 fatty acids, which have anti-inflammatory properties and support gut health. You can grill or bake salmon, flake it, and add it to your salads for a dose of healthy fats and protein.

Shrimp is a low-calorie and high-protein seafood option that can add a burst of flavor to your salads. It's also an excellent source of selenium, an antioxidant that supports immune function and protects against cellular damage.

Hard-boiled eggs are not only convenient but also provide a complete source of protein. They are rich in nutrients like vitamin B12 and choline, which are essential for brain health and metabolism.

You can use **Greek yogurt** as a creamy and protein-rich dressing or topping for salads. It's an excellent source of probiotics, calcium, and protein, which contribute to gut health and overall well-being.

Remember to choose organic, pasture-raised, or wild-caught options whenever possible to ensure the highest quality and nutritional value of the animal protein you incorporate into your salads. Pay attention to portion sizes and balance your animal protein with plenty of fresh vegetables, whole grains, and other gut-friendly ingredients.

By including these animal protein options in your salads, you can create a well-rounded and satisfying meal that supports your gut health while providing the nutrients your body needs.

Note: The quantities provided are for 2 medium size servings or one "Big Salad" serving. Adjust the portion sizes and ingredient amounts based on your desired taste, appetite, and weight loss goals.

Gut-Boosting Superfoods and Greens

1. Quinoa - Kale with Lemon Vinaigrette

- 2 cups chopped kale, stems removed
- 1 cup cooked red or white quinoa
- 1 small cucumber, diced
- 1 avocado, sliced
- 1/4 cup pomegranate seeds

- 1/4 cup chopped toasted walnuts
- Lemon vinaigrette dressing

Preparation:

1. Drizzle kale with olive oil and rub for 1 min to soften it. In a large mixing bowl, combine kale, quinoa, cucumber, and avocado.

2. Drizzle the lemon vinaigrette dressing over the salad and toss gently to coat.

3. Sprinkle with pomegranate seeds and chopped walnuts, and serve.

Lemon Vinaigrette Dressing

- 2 tablespoons fresh lemon juice
- 2 tablespoons extra-virgin olive oil
- 1 teaspoon Dijon mustard
- 1 garlic clove, minced
- Himalayan salt and pepper to taste

Preparation: In a small bowl, mix all ingredients until well combined.

2. Green and Purple Heaven

- 1 cup shredded green cabbage
- 1 cup shredded purple cabbage
- 1/2 cup green seedless grapes, halved
- 1/2 cup purple seedless grapes, halved

- 1 tablespoon pumpkin seeds
- 1 tablespoon sunflower seeds
- 1 tablespoon green onions, thinly sliced
- 1 tablespoon purple onion, finely chopped

Preparation: In a large mixing bowl, toss all ingredients. Add dressing and toss again.

Dressing:

- 1 tablespoon maple syrup
- 2 tablespoons extra virgin olive oil
- 1 tablespoon red wine vinegar
- 1 clove garlic, finely chopped
- Himalayan salt and pepper to taste

Preparation: In a small bowl, mix all ingredients until well combined.

3. Chickpea and Roasted Vegetables with Pomegranate Dressing

- 2 cups mixed salad greens (spinach, beet greens, radicchio, frisée, etc.)
- 1/2 cup roasted beets, sliced
- 1/2 cup roasted carrots, sliced
- 1 roasted red onion, quartered

- 1 cup cooked or canned chickpeas
- 1/3 cup crumbled feta cheese
- 2 tablespoons chopped fresh parsley
- 2 tablespoons chopped fresh mint
- 1 tablespoon extra virgin olive oil
- 1 tablespoon dried cranberries

Preparation:

1. Preheat the oven to 375 degrees Fahrenheit.

2. Wash and scrub beets and carrots, remove tops and bottoms; peel and quarter onion

3. Toss in olive oil, and roast for 45 min.

4. Drain the chickpeas, toss in olive oil, and roast for 20 min.

4. In a large salad bowl, combine cooled and sliced roasted beets, carrots, onions, chickpeas, and cranberries.

5. Drizzle with pomegranate dressing over the salad and toss gently to combine.

6. Put the tossed salad over mixed greens, and top with chopped fresh parsley, mint, and feta cheese.

Pomegranate Dressing

- 3 tablespoons pomegranate juice
- 2 tablespoons extra-virgin olive oil
- 1 tablespoon red wine vinegar

- 1 teaspoon honey
- 1/4 teaspoon ground cumin
- 1 garlic clove, minced
- Himalayan salt and pepper to taste

Preparation: In a small bowl, whisk together all ingredients until well combined.

4. Kale - Rapini Pecorino

- 1/4 bunch rapini
- 2 cups baby kale
- 1 lemon, juiced
- 1/3 cup grated Pecorino cheese
- 3 tablespoons extra virgin olive oil
- 2 garlic cloves, minced
- Himalayan salt and pepper to taste
- 1/2 teaspoon red chili flakes

Preparation:

1. Remove stems from rapini. Cut florets and leaves into medium size pieces.

2. Mix with baby kale.

3. Add dressing and toss until well combined.

4. Sprinkle with 1/ 2 Pecorino.

Dressing: In a bowl, whisk together lemon juice, olive oil, 1/2 Pecorino, garlic, salt and pepper until well combined.

5. Mediterranean Warm Bean Salad

- 2 cups baby arugula
- 1 cup cooked or canned white beans, drained
- 1 large Roma tomato
- 1/3 cup Kalamata olives
- 1 clove garlic, finely chopped
- 1 tablespoon basil pesto
- 1 tablespoon red onion, chopped
- 1 clove garlic, finely chopped
- 2 tablespoons extra virgin olive oil (1 for beans, 1 for dressing)
- 1 tablespoon lemon juice
- 1 tablespoon basil leaves, chopped
- 2 tablespoons alfalfa sprouts
- Himalayan salt and pepper to taste

Preparation:

1. Arrange arugula on a plate, then add chopped tomato and olives, and drizzle with olive oil and lemon juice.

2. Heat oil in a pan, add garlic and onions and saute for a few minutes until soft. Add white beans and cook until they are just warm.

3. Mix basil pesto into the bean mixture and toss until well combined.

4. Put bean mixture over arugula, and sprinkle with salt, pepper, alfalfa sprouts, and chopped basil leaves.

6. Warm Mushroom Hazelnut Salad

- 3 cups mixed salad greens (spinach, beet greens, radicchio, frisée, etc.)
- 2 cups assorted mushrooms (oyster, cremini, portobello, etc.) cleaned and chopped
- 2 tablespoons chopped fresh parsley
- 2 tablespoons sliced shallots
- 2 garlic cloves, chopped
- 2 tablespoons fresh thyme leaves, chopped
- 2 tablespoons extra virgin olive oil
- 1 tablespoon grass-fed butter
- 1/4 cup toasted hazelnuts
- Himalayan salt and pepper to taste

Preparation:

1. Heat a saute pan quickly over high heat, add olive oil and butter, add mushrooms, sprinkle with thyme, and season with salt and pepper.

2. Saute mushrooms for 5 minutes, stirring occasionally, until tender.

3. Add shallots and garlic and cook for 1-2 more minutes until slightly crispy.

4. In a large bowl, combine mixed greens and mushroom mixture. Add parsley, salt, pepper, and vinaigrette, and toss thoroughly.

5. Divide into 2 plates and top with hazelnuts.

Vinaigrette Dressing

- 2 tablespoons sherry vinegar
- 2 tablespoons extra-virgin olive oil
- 1 tablespoon finely minced shallots
- Himalayan salt and pepper to taste

Preparation: In a small bowl, whisk together all ingredients until well combined. Let sit for 10 minutes, then whisk olive oil.

7. Balsamic Tuna-Cantaloupe Salad

- 2 cups mixed salad greens (spinach, beet greens, radicchio, frisée, etc.)
- 1 cup cantaloupe, cubed
- 1 can tuna in water, drained and broken into chunks
- 2 tablespoons Cheddar cheese, grated
- 2 tablespoons fresh coriander, chopped
- 2 tablespoons balsamic vinegar

- 2 tablespoons extra virgin olive oil
- Himalayan salt and pepper to taste

Preparation:

1. In a bowl, mix tuna and cantaloupe. Add oil and vinegar, salt and pepper, and mix again.
2. Add mixed greens and toss gently.
3. Sprinkle with cheese and coriander, and serve.

Probiotic Powerhouses

8. Kimchi Potato Salad

- 1 cup new baby potatoes, boiled, cooled, and cubed
- 1 yam, baked and cubed
- 1/3 cup celery, chopped thinly and diagonally
- 1 tablespoon red onions, thinly sliced
- 1 tablespoon cilantro, chopped

Preparation:

1. In a large bowl, mix celery, onions, and cilantro with dressing.
2. Fold potatoes and yams gently and mix again.
3. Refrigerate before serving.

Dressing:

- 1/2 cup kimchi, with liquid
- 1 tablespoon maple syrup
- 2 tablespoons lime juice
- 2 tablespoons cold water
- 1 garlic clove, minced
- 1/2 red chili pepper, seeds removed, minced

Preparation: In a small bowl, whisk together all ingredients until well combined.

9. Fermented Beet and Cabbage Slaw

- 1/2 cup shredded red cabbage
- 1 cup shredded green cabbage
- 1 cup grated fermented beets
- 1/2 cup grated carrots
- 2 tablespoons green onions, thinly sliced
- 2 tablespoons raisins

Preparation:

1. Prepare the dressing first and set aside while preparing other ingredients.

2. In a mixing bowl, combine cabbage, beets, carrots, onions, and raisins.

3. Add dressing and toss the ingredients together until well combined, and serve.

Dressing:

- 2 tablespoons apple cider vinegar
- 1 tablespoon extra-virgin olive oil
- 1 tablespoon chopped fresh dill
- 1 tablespoon chopped fresh thyme
- 1 tablespoon maple syrup
- 1 teaspoon wholegrain mustard
- Himalayan salt and pepper to taste

Preparation: In a small bowl, combine all ingredients and mix well. Allow to sit for 10 minutes before adding to salad.

10. Probiotic Power Bowl

- 1 cup sauerkraut (live, refrigerated)
- 2 small beets
- 2 potatoes
- 2 carrots
- 1 cup canned white beans (drained, rinsed)
- 1/2 sweet onion
- 2 pickles (in brine, kosher)

- 1/2 English cucumber
- 1 small green apple, cored
- 2 tablespoons olive oil
- black pepper, to taste
- 2 tablespoons chopped dill and parsley

Preparation:

1. Steam or boil beets and carrots until tender. Bake or boil potatoes until cooked.

2. Put beets in cold water for a few minutes. When the beets are cool enough to handle, rub off the skin.

3. Cut the beets, carrots, pickles, cucumbers, apple, and potatoes into small cubes. Finely chop the onion.

4. In a large bowl, combine all ingredients, except for herbs and beets.

5. Add olive oil and mix all the ingredients well to ensure they are evenly coated.

6. Add beets and shopped herbs and mix again.

Serve the Probiotic Power Bowl as a main course for lunch or dinner. It is a perfect option for vegetarians and vegans looking for a nutritious and flavorful meal.

Growing up in Ukraine, this Probiotic Power Bowl was a beloved dish during the winter months when fresh green vegetables were not always available, but hearty root vegetables like beets, carrots, and potatoes were plentiful. The sauerkraut added a tangy and probiotic-rich element to this salad, making it a winter staple.

In Ukrainian cuisine, we believe it's important to incorporate fermented foods into our diet for their many health benefits. This salad has been a classic recipe passed down through generations.

Even though I now live in a different country, this salad holds a special place in my heart. It reminds me of cozy family gatherings and the warmth of home. As I share this recipe with you, I hope it brings the same joy to your table. Whether enjoyed during winter or any time of the year, this Probiotic Power Bowl delightfully combines flavors, minerals, vitamins, and probiotics. It's a wholesome and satisfying dish that will nourish your body and delight your taste buds.

11. Kimchi-Kale Sesame Toss

- 3 cups chopped kale, stems removed
- 1 cup kimchi, chopped
- 1/4 cup sliced red onions
- 1/4 cup shredded carrots
- 2 tablespoons toasted sesame seeds
- 2 tablespoons extra virgin olive oil

Preparation:

1. Drizzle kale with olive oil and rub for 1 min to soften it. In a large salad bowl, combine kale, chopped kimchi, sliced red onions, and shredded carrots.

2. Drizzle the olive oil over the salad and toss gently to combine.

3. Sprinkle toasted sesame seeds on top, and serve.

12. Roasted Radicchio - Blue Cheese Salad

- 1 medium radicchio head, cored and cut in wedges
- 1/4 cup toasted walnuts
- 2 tablespoons chopped Italian parsley
- 1 tablespoon extra virgin olive oil
- 3 tablespoons balsamic vinegar
- 1/2 cup crumbled Danish Blue Cheese
- 1 teaspoon honey
- a pinch of red pepper flakes
- Himalayan salt and pepper to taste

Preparation:

1. Preheat oven to 400 degrees Fahrenheit.

2. Brush radicchio wedges with olive oil and season with salt and pepper. Roast for 10-12 minutes, until radicchio is slightly darkened.

3. In a saucepan, combine balsamic vinegar, honey, and red pepper flakes. Cook over medium heat, stirring, for 4-5 minutes until reduced in half but still liquid.

4. Place radicchio on a platter, drizzle with balsamic reduction, and sprinkle with blue cheese, parsley, and walnuts.

13. Tahini-Miso Pasta Salad

- 2 cups cooked and rinsed bean or lentil short-cut pasta, chilled

(penne, fusilli, elbow macaroni, farfalle, etc.)

- 1/3 cup celery, finely chopped
- 1/3 cup cucumbers, chopped
- 1/3 cup broccoli florets, slightly blanched and cut into bite-size pieces
- 1/2 cup black kale, torn into small pieces
- 1/3 cup pickled carrots, chopped
- 2 tablespoons sunflower seeds

Preparation:

1. In a large salad bowl, combine all ingredients and mix well.

2. Chill in refrigerator for 30 min.

2. Add the Tahini-Miso dressing just before serving and toss until evenly coated.

Tahini-Miso Dressing

- 2 tablespoons sesame tahini
- 2 tablespoons sesame oil
- 1 tablespoon rice vinegar
- 1 tablespoon white miso paste
- 1 teaspoon honey
- pinch of chili flakes

Preparation: In a small bowl, combine all ingredients and mix well. Dress pasta salad just before serving.

14. Miso Tuna Salad Bites

- 1 can of tuna in water, drained
- 1 teaspoon miso
- 1 teaspoon rice vinegar
- 1/2 teaspoon honey
- 1 tablespoon avocado mayo
- Himalayan salt and pepper to taste
- 1 green onion, thinly sliced
- 1/2 avocado, sliced
- 3 mini cucumbers, sliced
- 1/2 package roasted seaweed snack
- 1 teaspoon sesame seeds

Preparation:

1. Mix tuna, mayo, miso, rice vinegar, honey, salt, and pepper.

2. Arrange cucumber and avocado slices on roasted seaweed, top with tuna mixture, and sprinkle with green onions and sesame seeds.

Hormone-Friendly Combos

15. Millet Supersalad

- 1 small purple sweet potato, peeled and cubed
- 1 small yam, peeled and cubed
- 1/2 cup cooked millet
- 1/2 cup canned chickpeas, drained
- 2 cups baby spinach or baby arugula
- 2 tablespoons extra-virgin olive oil
- 2 tablespoons sunflower seeds sprouts
- 1/2 teaspoon chili powder
- Himalayan salt and pepper to taste

Preparation:

1. Preheat oven to 400 degrees Fahrenheit.

2. In a bowl, mix yams and sweet potatoes with olive oil, salt, pepper, and chili powder.

3. Spread evenly on a baking sheet and bake for 25 minutes.

4. Mix millet, chickpeas, and baked veggies in a bowl with 1/2 dressing.

5. Arrange on a plate, sprinkle with sunflower seeds sprouts, and drizzle with the rest of the dressing.

Dressing:

- 2 tablespoons extra-virgin olive oil
- 2 tablespoons apple cider vinegar

- 1 teaspoon maple syrup
- 1 teaspoon Dijon mustard
- 1 garlic clove, minced

Preparation: In a small bowl, whisk all ingredients until well combined.

16. Herby Pistachio Smoked Salmon

- 3 cups mixed salad greens (spinach, beet greens, radicchio, frisée, etc.)
- 4 slices smoked wild Sockeye salmon, torn into small pieces
- 1 avocado, sliced
- 1 tablespoon extra virgin olive oil
- 2 teaspoons capers
- 1 tablespoon red onion, finely chopped
- 2 tablespoons pistachio, coarsely ground
- 1/4 cup green peas, fresh, or frozen and blanched

Preparation:

1. Heat oil in a small pan and fry capers for 2 minutes on high heat until crisp. Remove and drain on a paper towel.

2. Prepare dressing and set aside.

3. Divide greens on 2 plates and arrange smoked salmon and avocado slices on top.

4. Add green peas and red onions.

5. Drizzle with dressing and sprinkle with pistachios and crispy capers.

Herb Medley Dressing

- 1/2 cup avocado mayo
- 2 tablespoons lemon juice
- 1/2 cup herbs: tarragon, parsley, and chives
- Himalayan salt and pepper to taste

Preparation: Blend all ingredients in a blender until smooth.

17. Moroccan Roasted Cauliflower Walnut Date Crumble

- 2 cups baby spinach
- 1/2 cup chopped fresh parsley
- 2 cups cauliflower florets
- 1/4 cup walnuts, toasted
- 2 large dates, pitted
- 2 tablespoons hemp hearts
- 2 tablespoons pumpkin seeds, toasted
- 2 tablespoons extra-virgin olive oil
- 1 teaspoon ground cumin
- 1 lemon, juiced

- 1 garlic bulb
- Himalayan salt and pepper to taste

Preparation:

1. Preheat oven to 400 degrees Fahrenheit.

2. Put cauliflower into a bowl, add olive oil, cumin, salt, pepper, cumin, and mix until well combined.

3. Cut to top off the garlic bulb, sprinkle with olive oil, and wrap in foil.

4. Spread cauliflower evenly onto a baking tray. Bake cauliflower stirring occasionally, and garlic bulb, for 40 minutes.

5. In the meantime, roughly chop walnuts, pumpkin seeds, and dates. Add hemp hearts and parsley and continue to chop and mix until the crumble is textured and well combined.

6. Arrange spinach on a serving platter, drizzle with olive oil, and top with baked cauliflower.

7. Squeeze garlic cloves on top, drizzle with lemon juice, and sprinkle with walnut-date crumble.

18. Sesame Chicken Salad

- 1 chicken breast, baked or grilled, and shredded
- 1 carrot, julienned
- 1 cup red cabbage, shredded
- 1/4 cup edamame beans
- 2 tablespoons roasted cashews, coarsely ground

- 2 tablespoons cilantro leaves, chopped
- 1/4 cup yellow bell peppers, thinly sliced

Preparation: Mix all ingredients in a large bowl, add dressing, and mix again until evenly coated.

Dressing:

- 2 tablespoons extra virgin olive oil
- 1 teaspoon sesame oil
- 1 teaspoon soy sauce
- 1 teaspoon sesame seeds (black or white)
- chili flakes to taste
- 1 teaspoon honey
- 1 teaspoon rice vinegar

Preparation: In a small bowl, mix all ingredients until well combined.

19. Colorful Quinoa and Edamame with Ginger Soy Dressing

- 1/2 cup cooked white quinoa
- 1/2 cup cooked red quinoa
- 1 cup cooked edamame, shelled
- 1/2 cup diced bell peppers (assorted colors)
- 1/4 cup chopped fresh cilantro

- 2 tablespoons sliced green onions
- 2 tablespoons mung bean sprouts

Preparation:

1. In a mixing bowl, combine cooked quinoa, shelled edamame, diced bell peppers, and sliced green onions.

2. Drizzle the ginger soy dressing over the salad and toss gently to combine.

3. Divide the salad into two bowls or plates, sprinkle with chopped fresh cilantro, and mung bean sprouts, and serve.

Ginger Soy Dressing

- 1 tablespoon soy sauce
- 2 tablespoons rice vinegar
- 1 tablespoon sesame oil
- 1 tablespoon honey
- 1 teaspoon freshly grated ginger
- 1 garlic clove, minced

Preparation: In a small bowl, whisk together all ingredients until well combined.

20. Jicama - Turnip Curry Slaw

- 1 medium turnip, scrubbed and julienned
- 1 small jicama, peeled and julienned

- 1 medium carrot, shredded
- 1 medium apple, julienned
- 3 tablespoons unsalted sunflower seeds
- 1/2 cup silken tofu
- 1 teaspoon curry powder
- 1 tablespoon apple cider vinegar
- 3 garlic cloves, chopped
- 2 tablespoons coriander, chopped
- Himalayan salt and pepper to taste

Preparation:

1. Combine turnip, carrot, jicama, apple, and sunflower seeds.

2. In a blender, mix together tofu, curry powder, apple cider vinegar, garlic, salt, and pepper until smooth.

3. Mix salad with the tofu mixture until evenly coated.

4. Sprinkle with chopped coriander.

21. Warm and Cozy Red Cabbage Salad

- 1 tablespoon extra virgin olive oil
- 1 tablespoon grass-fed butter
- 1/2 sweet onion, sliced
- 2 garlic cloves, minced

- 1/2 small head of red cabbage, cored and shredded
- 2 tablespoons apple cider vinegar
- 1 orange, juiced
- 2 tablespoons golden raisins
- 2 tablespoons pumpkin seeds
- 2 tablespoons curly parsley, chopped
- Himalayan salt and pepper to taste

Preparation:

1. In a large cast iron pan, heat olive oil over medium heat. Add onion and saute for 5 min.

2. Reduce heat and add butter, garlic, and cabbage. Saute for 5 min.

3. Add apple cider vinegar, orange juice, salt and pepper, and raisins. Cook for 10 minutes, stirring occasionally, until the cabbage is soft and the liquid is gone. Remove from heat and let cool down.

4. Drizzle with tahini dressing and sprinkle with pumpkin seeds and parsley.

Tahini Dressing

- 1 tablespoon tahini
- 1 tablespoon whole-grain mustard
- 1 garlic clove, minced
- 1 tablespoon lemon juice

- Himalayan salt and pepper to taste

Preparation: In a small bowl, mix all ingredients until well combined and creamy.

22. Greek-Inspired Salad with Sardines

- 1 can of sardines in water, drained
- 1/4 cup sliced almonds, toasted
- 2 cups chopped kale or Romaine lettuce
- 1/2 cup cherry or Campari tomatoes, chopped
- 1/2 cucumber, peeled and sliced
- 1/4 cup pomegranate seeds
- 1/4 cup Kalamata olives, pitted
- 1/2 cup steamed small broccoli florets, cooled
- 1/2 cup canned white beans, rinsed and drained
- 1/4 cup crumbled goat feta cheese
- fresh oregano, chopped

Preparation:

1. Drizzle kale with olive oil and rub for 1 min to soften it. In a large mixing bowl, combine toasted almonds, chopped kale (or Romaine lettuce), tomatoes, cucumber, pomegranate seeds, olives, steamed broccoli, and beans.

2. Drizzle the dressing over the salad ingredients in the large bowl and gently toss to coat everything evenly.

3. Divide the salad into two serving bowls or plates.

4. Garnish with sardines and sprinkle feta cheese and oregano.

Dressing:

- 3 tablespoons extra-virgin olive oil
- 1 tablespoon red wine vinegar
- 1/2 teaspoon Dijon mustard
- 1 small garlic clove, minced
- Himalayan salt and pepper to taste

Preparation: In a small bowl, whisk together all ingredients until well combined.

Anti-inflammatory Bowls

23. Very Berry Spinach with Toasted Almonds

- 4 cups baby spinach
- 1 cup fresh mixed berries (strawberries, blueberries, raspberries)
- 1/4 cup toasted almonds
- 2 tablespoons crumbled goat cheese
- 2 tablespoons broccoli sprouts

- Himalayan salt and pepper to taste

Preparation:

1. In a large bowl, combine mixed berries and toasted almonds.

2. Drizzle the raspberry vinaigrette dressing over the salad mixture and toss gently to coat.

3. Add baby spinach and toss again.

3. Divide the salad into two bowls or plates, top with goat cheese and broccoli sprouts, and serve.

Raspberry Vinaigrette Dressing

- 3 tablespoons fresh or frozen raspberries
- 2 tablespoons extra-virgin olive oil
- 2 tablespoons red wine vinegar
- 1/2 teaspoon Dijon mustard
- 2 tablespoons diced shallots
- Himalayan salt and pepper to taste

Preparation: In a food processor, blend all ingredients for 30 sec on medium speed until well combined.

24. Minty Papaya Salad

- 1 cup ripe papaya, cubed
- 1/2 cup avocado, sliced
- 1/2 cup red bell peppers, sliced

- 2 tablespoons red onions, thinly sliced
- 1 tablespoon Goji berries
- 2 tablespoons fresh mint leaves
- 1 tablespoon hemp hearts

Preparation:

1. In a bowl, mix papaya, avocado, bell peppers, Goji berries, and onions
2. Drizzle with dressing, mix again, then sprinkle with chopped mint and hemp hearts

Dressing:

- 1 tablespoon extra virgin olive oil
- 2 tablespoons lime juice
- 1 pinch of Himalayan salt

Preparation: In a small bowl, mix all ingredients until well combined.

25. Fennel Apple Pecan

- 1/2 medium fennel bulb
- 1 cup baby spinach
- 1 medium green apple
- 1 celery stalk
- 1/3 cup roasted pecans

Preparation:

1. Thinly slice fennel and apple using a mandoline. Chop celery diagonally into small pieces.

2. Put the fennel, apple, and celery in a bowl, add dressing, and mix until evenly coated.

3. Add baby spinach and toss again.

4. Divide into 2 portions and top with roasted pecans.

Dressing:

- 2 tablespoons extra virgin olive oil
- 1 tablespoon orange juice
- 1 tablespoon lemon juice
- 1 teaspoon Dijon mustard
- Himalayan salt and pepper to taste

Preparation: In a small bowl, combine all ingredients and whisk together until well blended.

26. Arugula Pesto Pasta Salad

- 3 cups arugula
- 2 cups chickpea or bean short-cut pasta, cooked and cooled
- 2 tablespoons sun-dried tomatoes, soaked and chopped
- 1/4 cup roasted hazelnuts, chopped
- 2 tablespoons Italian parsley, chopped
- 3 garlic cloves, chopped

- 3 tablespoons extra virgin olive oil
- juice and zest of 1 lemon
- Himalayan salt and pepper to taste

Preparation:

1. In a food processor, combine arugula, garlic, lemon juice and zest, salt and pepper, and blend until all ingredients are broken down. While continuing to blend, slowly pour olive oil, and blend until very smooth.

2. Mix pasta, sun-dried tomatoes, and pesto until evenly coated.

3. Divide between plates and sprinkle with chopped hazelnuts and parsley. Serve at room temperature.

27. Mediterranean Parmigiano Oregano

- 2 cups Romaine lettuce, chopped
- 1/2 small radicchio
- 1/2 cup cooked or canned white kidney beans, drained
- 1/2 cup cherry tomatoes, halved
- 1/3 cup canned artichoke hearts, drained and chopped
- 1/4 cup pitted and sliced Kalamata olives
- 2 tablespoons red onions, thinly sliced
- 1/3 cup Parmigiano Reggiano cheese, grated
- 2 pepperoncini peppers, stemmed and thinly sliced

- 2 tablespoons broccoli sprouts
- 1 tablespoon pine nuts
- 3 pieces of sun-dried tomatoes, soaked and chopped

Preparation:

1. In a large salad bowl, combine all ingredients and toss until well mixed, adding Parmesan at the end.

2. Drizzle the Lemon Oregano dressing over the salad, and toss gently to coat. Top with broccoli sprouts.

Lemon Oregano Dressing

- 2 tablespoons fresh lemon juice
- 2 tablespoons extra-virgin olive oil
- 1 tablespoon fresh oregano, finely chopped
- 1 tablespoon shallots, finely chopped
- 1 garlic clove, minced
- Himalayan salt and pepper to taste

Preparation: In a small bowl, whisk together all ingredients until well combined.

28. Detoxifying Fruit Salad

- 1/2 cup mixed berries (blueberries, strawberries, raspberries)
- 1 orange, segmented

- 1/2 cup pineapple chunks
- 1/4 cup pitted cherries, chopped
- 1 tablespoon chopped almonds
- 1 tablespoon chopped walnuts
- 1 tablespoon chia seeds
- fresh mint leaves, for garnish

Preparation:

1. In a medium-sized bowl, combine the mixed berries, orange segments, pineapple chunks, and chopped cherries.

2. Pour the dressing over the fruit mixture and gently toss to coat the fruits evenly.

3. Sprinkle the chopped nuts and chia seeds.

4. Garnish with fresh mint leaves, and serve.

Dressing:

- 1/2 tablespoon freshly squeezed lemon juice
- 1/2 tablespoon freshly squeezed orange juice
- 1/2 tablespoon honey or maple syrup
- 1/4 teaspoon grated ginger
- a pinch of ground cinnamon

Preparation: In a separate small bowl, whisk together all ingredients until well combined.

29. Tangy Dandelion Detox

- 2 cups dandelion greens, chopped
- 1 cup thinly sliced Swiss chard
- 1 cup cooked farro
- 1/2 cup sliced cucumber
- 1/4 cup chopped fresh parsley
- 2 tablespoons hemp hearts
- 2 tablespoons radish sprouts

Preparation:

1. In a large bowl, combine the dandelion greens, Swiss chard, farro, sliced cucumber, chopped parsley, and hemp hearts.

2. Drizzle the dressing over the salad and toss to combine. Top with radish sprouts.

Dressing:

- 2 tablespoons apple cider vinegar
- 1 tablespoon Dijon mustard
- 1 tablespoon maple syrup
- 2 tablespoons extra-virgin olive oil
- Himalayan salt and pepper to taste

Preparation: In a small bowl, whisk together all ingredients until well combined.

30. Arugula Salad with Maitake Mushrooms and Parmesan

- 1 1/2 cups Maitake mushrooms, chopped
- 2 tablespoons onion, chopped
- 2 tablespoons extra virgin olive oil
- 2 garlic cloves, minced
- 1/2 cup cooked brown rice
- 1/2 cup cooked wild rice
- 2 cups baby arugula
- 1/2 lemon, juiced
- 2 tablespoons dried Goji berries
- 2 tablespoons walnuts, chopped and toasted
- 2 tablespoons Parmigiano Reggiano, grated
- Himalayan salt and pepper to taste

Preparation:

1. In a large cast iron pan, heat olive oil over medium heat. Add onions and garlic and saute for 5 min until soft.
2. Add mushrooms, mix well, and saute for 4 more min until mushrooms begin to cook but still firm.

3. Add lemon juice, rice and Goji berries, salt and pepper, mix again, and cook for 2 more minutes.

4. Divide arugula into two serving bowls or plates, drizzle with olive oil, and top with mushroom-rice mixture.

5. Sprinkle with Parmigiano and walnuts, and serve.

After refreshing salads for lunch, let's cozy up with some comforting and wholesome soups for dinner. As the day winds down, there's nothing quite like a nourishing bowl of soup to soothe the soul and fuel the body.

In the next chapter, we will dive into the world of soups, exploring a variety of recipes that are both satisfying and supportive of your gut health journey. From hearty vegetable soups to creamy purees, we will explore different textures, flavors, and ingredients that will leave you feeling nourished and satisfied.

Whether you're seeking a light and refreshing cold soup or a hearty and filling hot option, these recipes will offer you a range of choices to suit your taste preferences and dietary needs. They incorporate the principles we've learned about gut health, nutrient-dense ingredients, and the power of herbs and spices to create soups to contribute to your good health.

5

Evening Comfort: Soup Recipes

Benefits of Soups for Gut Health

Growing up in Ukraine, soups always held a special place in my family as well as all the families I knew. It seemed that no matter where you went, soups were a constant presence on the menu, whether for lunch or dinner. I have vivid memories of my Grandma preparing pots of steaming soups, emphasizing the importance of their gut-nourishing qualities.

In those days, the connection between soups and gut health wasn't widely discussed, but my Grandma intuitively understood their benefits long before it became a popular topic of conversation. Reflecting back, I realize that my Grandma's wisdom was ahead of its time. She instinctively recognized the nurturing and nourishing power of soups for our digestive system. Through the cooking traditions in our family, I developed a deep appreciation for the comforting and healing properties of soups.

Now, as I continue my journey of exploring the intricate relationship between food and gut health, I find solace in the familiar embrace of a steaming bowl of soup. It's a beautiful reminder of my roots and the wisdom passed down through generations. [30].

Benefits of Soups for Our Digestive System

One of the remarkable benefits of soups lies in their ability to facilitate easy digestion and enhance nutrient absorption. The liquid nature of soups promotes optimal digestion by "predigesting" the food outside of our bodies. By simmering ingredients in liquid for extended periods, soups break down tough fibers and release valuable nutrients. This process allows our digestive system to process the ingredients more efficiently.

Staying adequately hydrated is crucial for maintaining a healthy gut. Soups, with their high water content, play a significant role in keeping us hydrated. As we consume soups, we not only nourish our bodies with essential nutrients but also provide the hydration necessary for optimal digestive function.

Proper hydration supports the smooth movement of food through the digestive tract, aiding in regular bowel movements and preventing constipation. Additionally, a well-hydrated gut helps to maintain the integrity of the intestinal lining, ensuring proper absorption of nutrients and preventing the accumulation of harmful toxins.

Soups often include ingredients rich in electrolytes, such as potassium and sodium, which further contribute to maintaining a healthy fluid balance and supporting the optimal function of our gut.

By incorporating soups into our meals, we can enjoy the dual benefits of easy digestion and hydration, ensuring that our gut remains nourished and in optimal condition.

Broth to Support Gut Lining Repair

Vegetable Broth

Vegetable broth serves as a versatile and nourishing foundation for a wide array of soup recipes. This flavorful liquid, derived from simmering a variety of vegetables, herbs, and spices, provides not only a delicious base but also a host of benefits for our overall health. Vegetable broth is packed with essential nutrients, vitamins, and minerals, making it a nutritious addition to any soup. It is a fantastic option for those following a vegetarian or vegan diet, as it offers a plant-based alternative to meat-based broths. With its comforting flavors and numerous health benefits, vegetable broth takes your soups to a whole new level of nourishment and satisfaction.

Homemade Vegetable Broth Recipe

- 3 carrots, roughly chopped
- 2 celery stalks, roughly chopped
- 1 onion, roughly chopped
- 4 garlic cloves, smashed
- 1 leek, roughly chopped
- 1 parsnip, roughly chopped
- 1 beet, roughly chopped
- 1 bunch of fresh parsley
- 2 bay leaves
- 1/2 teaspoon peppercorns

- 10 cups filtered water

Preparation:

1. In a large pot or a slow cooker, combine all the ingredients: carrots, celery, onion, garlic, leek, parsnip, beet, parsley, bay leaves, and peppercorns.

2. Pour water into the pot, ensuring that the vegetables are fully covered.

3. Place the pot over medium-high heat and bring to a boil.

4. Reduce the heat to low and simmer for 1 minimum hour. Or simmer for 8-12 hours if using a slow cooker.

5. Remove from heat and strain the broth into a separate container, discarding the cooked vegetables and herbs.

6. Allow the broth to cool before storing it in airtight containers in the refrigerator or freezer.

You can customize the flavor of the vegetable broth by adding additional herbs or spices according to your taste preferences. Feel free to experiment with ingredients like thyme, rosemary, ginger, or turmeric to enhance the nutritional profile and add extra depth of flavor to your broth.

Enjoy this nourishing and gut-supportive vegetable broth as a foundation for your soups, or simply sip it on its own for a comforting and gut-supportive drink providing a soothing and healing experience for your gut lining repair.

The Magic of Bone Broth

Bone broth has been honored as a powerful elixir for gut health, offering many benefits that extend far beyond its flavor. This nourishing liquid is rich in essential nutrients, amino acids, collagen, and gelatin, all of which play a crucial role in supporting a healthy gut lining and promoting overall wellness.

One of the key benefits of bone broth is its potential to heal and repair a leaky gut. Leaky gut syndrome is a condition where the lining of the intestines becomes permeable, allowing harmful substances to leak into the bloodstream. The gelatin and collagen found in bone broth provide the building blocks for repairing and restoring the integrity of the gut lining, helping to seal the gaps and prevent further "leakage".

Additionally, bone broth is a fantastic source of amino acids such as glutamine and glycine, which are known to have anti-inflammatory properties. These amino acids help to reduce inflammation in the gut, soothing and calming the digestive system. The gelatin in bone broth also supports the growth of beneficial bacteria in the gut, contributing to a healthy and balanced gut microbiome.

Incorporating bone broth into your daily diet is easy. It can be enjoyed as a warming and comforting drink on its own or used as a base for soups, stews, sauces, and even as a cooking liquid for grains and legumes. By substituting water or store-bought broth with homemade bone broth, you can infuse your meals with its rich flavors and exceptional nutritional profile.

Homemade Bone Broth Recipe

Making your own bone broth at home is a simple process. By using high-quality bones from organic, pasture-raised animals, you can ensure that your broth is free from harmful additives and rich in nutrients.

- 2-3 pounds of organic, pasture-raised beef or chicken bones

- 1 onion, chopped
- 1 leek, chopped
- 3 carrots, chopped
- 2 celery stalks, chopped
- 4 cloves of garlic, smashed
- a handful of fresh herbs such as parsley, thyme, or rosemary
- 2 tablespoons of apple cider vinegar
- 10 cups filtered water

Preparation:

1. Preheat your oven to 400 degrees Fahrenheit. Place the bones on a baking sheet and roast them for 30 minutes to enhance their flavor.

2. Transfer the roasted bones to a large stockpot or a slow cooker. Add the chopped vegetables, garlic, herbs, and apple cider vinegar.

3. Fill the pot with enough filtered water to cover the bones and vegetables.

4. Bring the mixture to a boil, then reduce the heat to low and simmer for at least 8 hours, or up to 24 hours in a slow cooker for maximum flavor and nutrient extraction. Skim off any foam or impurities that rise to the surface.

5. Strain the broth through a fine-mesh sieve or cheesecloth into a container. Discard the solids.

6. Allow the broth to cool before transferring it to the refrigerator or freezer for storage. The fat may solidify on top, which can be removed if desired.

By incorporating bone broth into your daily meals and enjoying its nourishing properties, you can promote gut health, support healing, and contribute to your overall well-being. Experiment with different variations and recipes to find the flavors and combinations that resonate with you.

Steamy Hugs for Your Gut: Hot Soups

Note: The quantities provided are for 4 medium size servings. Adjust the portion sizes and ingredient amounts based on your desired consistency, taste, weight loss goals, and appetite.

1. Gingery Carrot Soup

- 1 tablespoon coconut oil
- 1 teaspoon cumin seeds
- 1 teaspoon ground cumin
- 1 teaspoon turmeric
- 1 onion, diced
- 2 cloves garlic, minced
- 1-inch piece of ginger, grated
- 4 large carrots, peeled and chopped
- 4 cups vegetable broth

- 1 cup cooked wild rice
- 1 cup coconut milk
- 1 teaspoon apple cider vinegar
- Himalayan salt and pepper to taste
- 1 tablespoon fresh cilantro, chopped

Preparation:

1. Heat the coconut oil in a pot over medium heat. Add cumin seeds and saute for 1 min. Add onion, garlic, and ginger. Sauté until the onion is soft.

2. Add the sliced carrots, ground cumin, and turmeric and cook for a few minutes, stirring occasionally.

3. Pour in the vegetable broth and bring to a boil. Reduce the heat and simmer for about 15-20 minutes until the carrots are tender. Remove from heat and allow to cool down.

4. Blend the soup until smooth.

5. Return the soup to the pot and stir in the coconut milk, wild rice, and apple cider vinegar. Heat again until hot. Season with salt and pepper to taste, and more spices if desired.

6. Serve hot, garnished with fresh cilantro.

2. Curry Pumpkin Soup

- 1 tablespoon coconut oil
- 1 onion, chopped

- 2 cloves garlic, minced
- 2 cups cubed pumpkin
- 5 cups vegetable broth
- 1 teaspoon curry powder
- 1/2 teaspoon ground cinnamon
- Himalayan salt and pepper to taste
- 2 tablespoons coconut cream
- 2 tablespoons toasted pumpkin seeds

Preparation:

1. Heat the oil in a large pot over medium heat. Add the diced onion and minced garlic, and sauté until the onion becomes translucent.

2. Add the pumpkin to the pot and cook for a few minutes, stirring occasionally.

3. Pour in the vegetable broth and bring to a boil. Reduce the heat and simmer for about 25-30 minutes, or until the pumpkin is tender.

4. Remove from heat, allow to cool down, and blend the soup until smooth.

5. Return the soup to the pot and stir in curry powder and cinnamon, season with salt and pepper to taste, and heat again on low heat.

6. Drizzle with coconut cream, sprinkle with pumpkin seeds, and serve hot.

3. Lentil and Swiss Chard Soup

- 2 tablespoons extra virgin olive oil
- 1 onion, chopped
- 1 carrot, chopped
- 1 celery stalks, chopped
- 3 cloves of garlic, minced
- 1 cup dried red lentils, rinsed
- 1 cup canned tomatoes, drained and chopped
- 6 cups vegetable broth
- 1 bay leaf
- 1/2 teaspoon dried thyme
- 1 teaspoon ground cumin
- 1 teaspoon curry powder
- 1/2 teaspoon paprika
- 1 cup Swiss Chard leaves, chopped
- Himalayan salt and pepper to taste
- 1 lemon, juiced
- 2 tablespoons parsley, chopped

Preparation:

1. In a large pot, heat the olive oil over medium heat. Add the onion, carrot, celery, and garlic. Sauté until the vegetables are tender, about 5 minutes.

2. Add thyme, cumin, curry, and paprika. Cook for under 1 minute, stirring constantly.

3. Add tomatoes and cook for a few minutes, stirring often.

4. Add the rinsed lentils, vegetable broth, salt, pepper, and bay leaf to the pot. Stir to combine.

5. Bring the mixture to a boil slowly, then reduce the heat to low. Cover the pot and simmer for about 30 minutes, or until the lentils are cooked.

6. Add the chopped Swiss Chard to the pot. Stir well and simmer for an additional 5-10 minutes until the chard is soft and wilted.

7. Remove the bay leaf, and season with salt, pepper, and spices. Add lemon juice and stir well.

8. Sprinkle with chopped parsley and serve hot.

4. Cozy Pear - Fennel Soup

- 2 tablespoons coconut oil
- 2 leeks (white parts), chopped
- 1 fennel, cored and chopped
- 1 pear, cored and chopped
- 1/2 teaspoon dried thyme
- 1 tablespoon fresh thyme, chopped

- 1 teaspoon ground turmeric
- Himalayan salt and pepper to taste
- 5 cups vegetable broth
- 2 tablespoons toasted pumpkin seeds

Preparation:

1. In a large saucepan, heat the coconut oil over medium heat. Add chopped leeks and dried thyme and cook until leeks are softened.

2. Add chopped fennel and pear, mix well, and cook for a few more minutes. Add turmeric and mix well.

3. Add vegetable broth, salt and pepper, and bring to a boil.

4. Reduce heat and simmer for 10-15 minutes, stirring occasionally, until fennel and pear are soft.

5. Allow to cool down and puree in a blender until smooth. Warm up before serving and sprinkle with pumpkin seeds and fresh thyme.

5. Butternut Squash Soup with Stilton and Walnuts

- 1 teaspoon extra virgin olive oil
- 1 medium butternut squash, cut in half and seeded
- 1/4 cup crumbled Stilton
- 2 tablespoons toasted walnuts, coarsely chopped
- 1/2 teaspoon dried sage
- 1 tablespoon fresh sage, chopped

- Himalayan salt and pepper to taste
- 5 cups vegetable broth

Preparation:

1. Preheat oven to 375 degrees Fahrenheit. Rub squash with olive oil, wrap in foil, and bake for 45 - 60 min.

2. Remove squash from the oven, cool down, peel, and chop.

3. Put squash in a food processor, add dried sage, salt and pepper, and puree until smooth.

4. Transfer to a saucepan, stir with remaining broth, or to desired consistency, and simmer for 5-10 minutes.

5. Sprinkle with Stilton, fresh sage, and walnuts, and serve.

6. Golden Roots Soup

- 2 tablespoons coconut oil
- 1 small leek, white part, thinly sliced
- 1 small onion, chopped
- 2 cloves garlic, chopped
- 1 medium carrot, chopped
- 1/2 small rutabaga, chopped
- 1 small parsnip, chopped
- 1 medium turnip, chopped
- 1 small yam, chopped

- 4 cups vegetable broth
- 1 cup coconut milk
- 1 tablespoon tandoori spice (or mix your own with equal parts of ground cumin, ginger, cinnamon, coriander, turmeric, cardamom, and nutmeg)
- Himalayan salt and pepper to taste
- 2 tablespoons fresh cilantro, chopped

Preparation:

1. Heat the coconut oil in a pot over medium heat. Add onion, garlic, and leek. Sauté until soft.

2. Add all vegetables and vegetable broth. Make sure vegetables are covered with broth, add water if needed. Bring to a boil.

3. Reduce the heat, cover the pot, and simmer for about 30 minutes until vegetables are tender. Remove from heat and allow to cool down.

4. Blend the soup until smooth.

5. Return to the pot and stir in the coconut milk. Heat again until hot. Add more milk or water if it's too thick. Season with salt and pepper to taste, and more spice if desired.

6. Sprinkle with fresh cilantro and serve.

7. Earthy Cashew Mushroom Soup

- 1 cup raw cashews, soaked overnight and drained
- 2 tablespoons avocado oil

- 1 leek, white part, finely sliced
- 2 cloves garlic, chopped
- 1 small onion, chopped
- 1 medium potato, scrubbed and chopped
- 1 1/2 cups cremini mushrooms, chopped
- 5 cups vegetable broth
- 1 teaspoon rice vinegar
- 1 tablespoon fresh thyme leaves
- 1 fresh thyme sprig
- Himalayan salt and pepper to taste

Preparation:

1. Heat the avocado oil in a pot over medium heat. Add onion and leek. Sauté until soft.

2. Add garlic and mushrooms and saute for 5 min.

3. Add broth, vinegar, and thyme sprig, and bring to a boil.

4. Reduce the heat, cover the pot, and simmer for about 10 minutes. Remove from heat and discard the thyme sprig. Allow to cool down.

4. Blend the soup well until smooth and return to the pot.

5. Blend cashews with 2 cups of mushroom soup on high speed until fully blended and creamy.

6. Add the cashew mixture to the pot and heat the soup stirring occasionally so that cashew cream is fully mixed with the soup. Season with salt and pepper to taste.

7. Sprinkle with fresh thyme and serve.

8. Moroccan Tomato Soup

- 1 cup canned chickpeas, drained
- 2 tablespoons extra virgin olive oil
- 1 can diced tomatoes, in juice
- 2 cloves garlic, chopped
- 1 onion, chopped
- 1 celery stalk, chopped
- 1/2 teaspoon cinnamon
- 1/2 teaspoon turmeric
- 5 cups vegetable broth
- 2 tablespoons fresh parsley, chopped
- 2 tablespoons fresh cilantro, chopped
- 1 teaspoon fresh ginger, grated
- Himalayan salt and pepper to taste

Preparation:

1. Heat the avocado oil in a pot over medium heat. Add onion, garlic, celery, cinnamon, turmeric, and ginger. Sauté until soft.

2. Add chickpeas, tomatoes with juice, and vegetable broth and bring to a boil.

3. Reduce the heat, add salt and pepper to taste, cover the pot, and simmer for about 10 minutes.

4. Sprinkle with parsley and cilantro, and serve.

9. Sweet Roasted Sage Soup

- 2 lbs Roma tomatoes, quartered
- 1/2 cup extra virgin olive oil
- 1 whole garlic bulb, cloves separated
- 1 red onion, quartered
- 1 tablespoon maple syrup
- 1/2 cup sage leaves
- 1 can white beans, drained and rinsed
- 4 cups vegetable broth
- Himalayan salt and pepper to taste

Preparation:

1. Preheat oven to 400 degrees Fahrenheit. Mix maple syrup with 1/2 of olive oil in a small bowl.

2. Put tomatoes, garlic, and onion into a roasting pan and pour the maple syrup mixture over it. Mix well to coat vegetables evenly. Roast for 45 min until tomatoes are soft.

3. In the meantime, heat the remaining oil over medium heat and fry sage leaves, stirring occasionally, for 1-2 min, until crisp. Remove, drain the leaves, and save the oil.

4. Remove vegetables from the oven and peel garlic. Allow to cool down and then blend coarsely until well mixed, but not smooth.

5. Pour into a pot, add beans and vegetable broth, and cook on medium heat until hot, stirring occasionally.

5. Sprinkle with fried sage leaves and sage-infused olive oil, and serve.

10. Roasted Buckwheat Mushroom Soup

- 1/3 cup roasted buckwheat
- 2 tablespoons extra virgin olive oil
- 1 onion, chopped
- 1 medium carrot, chopped
- 4 cloves garlic, chopped
- 4 oyster mushrooms, chopped
- 2 celery stalks, chopped
- 1 teaspoon dried oregano
- 1 teaspoon dried dill
- 2 tablespoons fresh dill, chopped

- 2 tablespoons fresh parsley, chopped
- 2 bay leaves
- 2 medium potatoes, scrubbed and cubed
- 6 cups vegetable broth
- Himalayan salt and pepper to taste

Preparation:

1. If using raw buckwheat, toast it on a dry pan over medium heat for 5 min stirring continuously, until golden brown.

2. In a pot, heat oil on medium heat, add celery, carrots, onion, mushrooms, garlic, dried oregano, and dill, and saute for 5 min.

3. Add rinsed buckwheat, potatoes, bay leaves, salt, and vegetable broth. Bring to a boil, cover, and cook for 15-20 min on medium heat.

4. Sprinkle with pepper, fresh dill, and parsley, and serve.

11. Classic Vegetarian Ukrainian Borsch

It's my cherished Borsch recipe. As I stood by my Grandmother's side in the kitchen, I learned the secrets of creating this beloved soup. But as time passed, I found my own healthy cooking path. While my grandmother's traditional and very tasty Ukrainian borsch was laden with hearty meats and lard, I've taken a different route, crafting a vegetarian version that aligns with my own preferences. It's a blend of heritage and individuality, a tribute to my past, and a nod to my new healthy lifestyle. Each spoonful carries the flavors of beets, cabbage, and lots of garlic, and the essence of a family history that bridges generations.

- 3 medium scrubbed yellow potatoes, cubed

- 1 onion, chopped
- 2 medium carrots, chopped
- 6 cloves garlic, chopped
- 1 medium beet, scrubbed
- 3 cups green cabbage, shredded
- 1 cup beet greens, chopped
- 2 celery stalks, chopped
- 1 sweet red pepper, sliced
- 1 can kidney beans, drained and rinsed
- 1/3 cup chopped fresh dill
- 1/3 cup chopped fresh parsley
- 1/4 cup olive oil
- 1/2 can tomato paste or 1 can tomato sauce
- 1/4 cup sour cream or Greek yogurt
- 8 cups vegetable broth

Preparation:

1. Steam the beets until soft, put in cold water for a few minutes, and peel the skin off. Slice in matchsticks using a mandoline slicer.

2. Heat the oil in a large pot over medium heat. Add onion, 1/2 garlic, and sauté until soft, for 5 min.

3. Add carrots and celery and saute for 5 more min.

4. Add tomato paste or tomato sauce, stir well, and saute for 5 more minutes, stirring occasionally.

5. Add potatoes, cabbage, beet greens, and broth, and bring to a boil.

6. Reduce the heat, cover the pot, and simmer for about 10 minutes. Add sweet peppers, beans, and beets. Simmer for 10-15 more minutes, stirring occasionally.

7. Season with salt and pepper, add dill, parsley, and the remaining garlic. Simmer for 1 more minute and remove from heat.

8. Serve with a spoonful of sour cream or Greek yogurt and a generous sprinkle of fresh dill.

12. Salmon and Brown Rice Soup

- 2 cups cooked brown rice
- 2 cans of Wild Alaskan Salmon
- 2 tablespoons avocado oil
- 1 small yellow onion, chopped
- 2 cloves garlic, chopped
- 6 cups vegetable broth
- 2 yellow potatoes, scrubbed and cubed
- 2 green onions, thinly sliced
- 1 tablespoon soy sauce

- 1 tablespoon chopped fresh dill
- 1 tablespoon chopped fresh parsley
- 1 tablespoon chopped fresh coriander
- 2 carrots, sliced
- 1 tablespoon fresh ginger, grated
- Himalayan salt and pepper to taste

Preparation:

1. Heat the avocado oil in a pot over medium heat. Add onion, garlic, ginger, and carrots. Sauté for a few minutes.

2. Add potatoes, cooked rice, and vegetable broth and bring to a boil. Reduce the heat, cover the pot, and cook until potatoes are soft, for 10-15 min.

3. In a bowl, break the canned salmon into medium-sized chunks, remove skin and bones, and mix with soy sauce.

4. Add salmon to soup, mix gently, and simmer for a few minutes for flavors to mingle. Add salt and pepper if needed.

5. Sprinkle with green onions, dill, parsley, and cilantro, and serve hot.

13. Herby Chicken Meatballs Soup

- 1 lb ground chicken breast
- 2 tablespoons extra virgin olive oil
- 1 egg, beaten

- 1 small yellow onion, chopped
- 4 cloves garlic, finely chopped
- 4 cups chicken or vegetable broth
- 2 yellow potatoes, scrubbed and cubed
- 2 green onions, thinly sliced
- 2 cups kale, stemmed and chopped
- 1/2 teaspoon dried dill
- 1/2 teaspoon dried oregano
- 1/2 teaspoon dried basil
- 1 tablespoon fresh parsley, chopped
- 1 carrot, sliced
- 2 celery stalks, sliced
- Himalayan salt and pepper to taste

Preparation:

1. In a large bowl, mix ground chicken, egg, grated onion, 1/2 garlic, dry herbs, salt and pepper. Make small balls using wet hands.

2. Heat the olive oil in a pot over medium heat. Add meatballs and fry for a few minutes until slightly browned.

3. Add chopped onion, 1/2 garlic, celery, and carrots. Sauté for a few minutes.

4. Add broth, potatoes, chopped kale, and vegetable or chicken broth and slowly bring to a boil.

5. Reduce the heat, add salt and pepper, cover the pot, and cook for 10-15 min.

6. Sprinkle with fresh parsley, and serve.

14. Split Pea Soup with Paprika and Almonds

- 2 tablespoons extra virgin olive oil
- 1 small yellow onion, chopped
- 4 cloves garlic, chopped
- 5 cups vegetable broth
- 2 green onions, thinly sliced
- 1 cup dry split peas, rinsed
- 1 teaspoon dried tarragon
- 1 teaspoon smoked paprika
- 2 tablespoons toasted sliced almonds
- 1 carrot, chopped
- 2 celery stalks, chopped
- Himalayan salt and pepper to taste

Preparation:

1. Heat the olive oil in a pot over medium heat. Add onion, tarragon, and garlic and sauté for a few minutes.

2. Add celery and carrot. Sauté for a few minutes.

3. Add peas and broth and bring to a boil.

4. Reduce heat, add salt and paprika, cover the pot, and simmer for 15 min until peas are cooked.

5. Sprinkle with more paprika, green onions, and toasted almonds, and serve.

15. Ginger - Almond Yam Soup

- 2 tablespoons coconut oil
- 1 small yellow onion, chopped
- 4 cloves garlic, chopped
- 1 can of coconut milk
- 2 cups vegetable broth
- 2 large yams
- 2 tablespoons fresh ginger, grated
- 2 tablespoons fresh coriander, chopped
- 1 teaspoon curry powder
- 1 teaspoon ground cumin
- 1 teaspoon cumin seeds

- 2 tablespoons smooth almond butter
- Himalayan salt to taste

Preparation:

1. Preheat the oven to 400 degrees Fahrenheit. Place yams on a baking sheet and bake for 45 min or until soft. Remove the skin.

2. Heat coconut oil in a pot over medium heat. Add onion, garlic, ginger, cumin seeds, cumin, curry powder, and sauté for a few minutes while stirring often. Allow to cool down.

3. Put yams in a blender, add vegetable broth and onion-garlic-ginger mixture, and blend until smooth.

4. Return blended yams to the pot, add coconut milk and salt, mix well and slowly bring to a boil. You will need to cover the pot during this time as the soup will "spit".

5. Mix in almond butter and simmer for 5 more min stirring often until almond butter is completely mixed and dissolved.

6. Sprinkle with fresh coriander, and serve.

16. Chicken Sauerkraut Soup

- 2 tablespoons extra virgin oil
- 1 small yellow onion, chopped
- 4 cloves garlic, chopped
- 2 cups canned sauerkraut
- 4 cups chicken or vegetable broth

- 1 chicken breast, baked and chopped
- 1 large carrot, sliced
- 2 yellow potatoes, scrubbed and cubed
- 1 bay leaf
- 2 tablespoons fresh dill, chopped

Preparation:

1. Heat the olive oil in a pot over medium heat. Add onion, garlic, and chicken, and fry for a few minutes until slightly browned.

2. Add potatoes, carrots, bay leaf, sauerkraut, and broth, and bring to a boil.

3. Reduce heat, cover the pot, and simmer the soup for about 30 min. Add salt if required, but it should be salty enough.

4. Sprinkle with black pepper and dill, and serve.

Refreshing Wellness: Cold Soups

Cold soups are not only delicious but refreshing – perfect for the hot weather. These cold soups are full of different flavors and textures that will make your taste buds happy. And there's a bonus that you won't find in hot soups. They're a perfect home for live probiotics that can't survive in hot soups, adding even more goodness to every spoonful.

Note: The quantities provided are for 4 medium size servings. Adjust the portion sizes and ingredient amounts based on your desired consistency, taste, weight loss goals, and appetite.

17. Red Ginger Summer Soup

- 2 tablespoons olive oil
- 1 red onion, diced
- 1 cup rhubarb, trimmed and chopped
- 2 cup beets, peeled and chopped
- 3 cloves of garlic, chopped
- 2 teaspoons fresh ginger, grated
- 2 teaspoons fresh dill, chopped
- 1 teaspoon ground cumin
- Himalayan salt and pepper to taste
- 4 cups vegetable broth
- 1/2 cup Greek yogurt
- 2 tablespoons fresh dill, chopped, for garnish

Preparation:

1. In a large saucepan, heat the olive oil over medium heat. Add the diced onion and cook until softened for 5- 10 min. Add garlic, ginger, and cumin and cook for 2 min.
2. Add beets and rhubarb, mix well, then add vegetable broth, salt and pepper, and bring to a boil.
3. Reduce heat and simmer for 30-40 minutes, stirring occasionally, until beets are soft.

4. Allow to cool down and blend until smooth. Serve with a dollop of yogurt and a sprinkle of dill.

18. Zucchini-Parmesan Sunshine Soup

- 2 tablespoons extra virgin olive oil
- 2 medium yellow zucchini, chopped
- 2 cloves of garlic, chopped
- 1/2 cup grated Parmesan
- 2 tablespoons toasted almonds, coarsely chopped
- 1/2 ground almonds
- Himalayan salt and pepper to taste
- 4 cups vegetable broth

Preparation:

1. Dry-fry ground almonds on medium-low heat, stirring frequently, until golden brown.
2. In a large pot, saute garlic in olive oil on medium heat for a few minutes.
3. Add vegetable broth, zucchini, salt and pepper, bring to a boil, and cook for 20 min on medium heat.
4. Cool down, put into a blender, and blend until smooth.
5. Sprinkle with Parmesan and chopped almonds, and serve.

19. Crabby Avocado Soup

- 2 avocados, chopped
- 2 tablespoons avocado oil
- 1 cup yellow grape tomatoes
- 2 jalapeno peppers, seeds and membranes removed, chopped
- 2 cloves garlic, chopped
- 2 green onions, thinly sliced
- 1 small onion, chopped
- 2 tablespoons cilantro, chopped
- 2 tablespoons lime juice
- 1 can of crab meat
- 1 cup Greek yogurt
- 1 cup vegetable broth
- Himalayan salt and pepper to taste

Preparation:

1. Heat 1 tablespoon oil in a pan on medium heat, add tomatoes, garlic, 1/2 chopped jalapenos, and chopped onion, and saute for 15 min or until soft.
2. In the meantime, in a small bowl, mix the remaining jalapenos, green onions, 1 tablespoon of avocado oil, cilantro, salt/pepper, and flaked crab meat. Refrigerate until ready to serve.

3. Allow sauteed vegetables to cool down, add vegetable broth, avocados, yogurt, lime juice, salt and pepper, and blend well until smooth. Refrigerate until ready to serve.

4. Divide soup between bowls, top with crab mixture, and serve.

20. Cold Summer Okroshka

- 3 medium baked potatoes, cooled and cubed
- 2 green onions, thinly sliced
- 2 hard-boiled eggs, chopped
- 1/2 English cucumber, chopped
- 6 red radishes, thinly sliced
- 1/3 cup chopped fresh dill
- 1/3 cup chopped fresh parsley
- 4 cups of Kvass OR unsweetened Kefir
- 1 lemon, juiced
- 1/4 cup sour cream or Greek yogurt (if using Kvass for liquid)
- Himalayan salt and pepper to taste

Preparation:

1. Mix all chopped vegetables and divide between bowls.
2. Mix Kvass or Kefir with lemon juice.
3. Pour Kvass or Kefir over the mixture and generously sprinkle

with herbs, add salt and pepper.

4. If using Kvass, add a dollop of sour cream or Greek yogurt, and mix well.

21. Summer Ukrainian Borsch

- 3 medium scrubbed yellow potatoes, cubed
- 1 onion, chopped
- 2 bay leaves
- 2 medium carrots, chopped
- 4 cloves garlic, chopped
- 1 medium beet, scrubbed
- 2 cups green cabbage, shredded
- 2 celery stalks, chopped
- 1/2 sweet red pepper, sliced
- 1 can kidney beans, drained and rinsed
- 1/3 cup chopped fresh dill
- 1/3 cup chopped fresh parsley
- 2 tablespoons olive oil
- 1/2 can tomato paste or 1 can tomato sauce
- 1/4 cup Greek yogurt

- 8 cups vegetable broth
- 1 cup pickles in brine, chopped

Preparation:

1. Steam the beets until soft, put in cold water for a few minutes, and peel the skin off. Slice in matchsticks using a mandoline slicer.
2. Heat the broth in a large pot over medium heat. Add tomato paste or sauce and stir well until fully mixed. Add carrots, cabbage, and potatoes, bring to a boil, and cook on medium heat for 10-15 min.
3. Add celery, sweet peppers, and beans. Simmer for 10 more minutes, stirring occasionally.
4. Add onions, garlic, olive oil, beets, and herbs, season with salt and pepper, reduce the heat, and simmer for 2-3 more minutes.
5. Remove from heat, allow to cool down, and refrigerate until cold.
6. Serve with a spoonful of Greek yogurt, a tablespoon of chopped pickles, and a generous sprinkle of fresh dill.

22. Mango-Coconut Soup

- 2 cups cubed mango, either fresh or frozen and thawed
- 1 cup Greek yogurt
- 1 cup coconut milk
- 1 tablespoon lemon juice

- 1/2 teaspoon ground cinnamon
- mint leaves for garnish
- 1 teaspoon lemon zest for garnish

Preparation:

1. Combine all ingredients in a blender and blend until smooth.
2. Refrigerate for an hour.
3. Serve with mint and lemon zest garnish.

23. Cucumber Soup with Feta

- 1 English cucumber, peeled and chopped
- 1 cup Greek yogurt
- 1 cup vegetable broth
- 1 tablespoon lemon juice
- 2 tablespoons goat feta cheese, crumbled
- 4 tablespoons fresh dill, chopped
- 2 tablespoons green onions, chopped

Preparation:

1. Combine cucumber, yogurt, broth, lemon juice, and 1/2 dill in a blender and blend until smooth.
2. Refrigerate for an hour.

3. Sprinkle with feta cheese, black pepper, 1/2 dill, and green onions, and serve

24. Green Goddess Gazpacho

- 1 cup frozen green peas
- 2 cups spinach
- 1 large bunch of asparagus
- 2 cups vegetable broth
- 1 tablespoon lemon juice
- 2 tablespoons olive oil
- 2 tablespoons Greek yogurt
- 1/2 avocado
- 1 leek, white part only, chopped
- 1 jalapeno pepper, seeds and membranes removed, chopped
- 2 garlic cloves, minced
- 1/4 cup fresh tarragon, chopped, and a pinch for garnish
- Himalayan salt and pepper to taste

Preparation:

1. Cut the "woody" ends from the asparagus stalks and discard. Cut the tips and save. Cut the rest of the asparagus into 1-inch pieces.

2. In a large pot, heat olive oil on medium heat, add leek, jalapeno, tarragon, and garlic, and saute for 5 min until soft.
3. Add asparagus and cook for 4 min or until tender. Add spinach, mix well, and cook until wilted.
4. Add vegetable broth and peas, bring to a boil, and cook until peas are fully defrosted.
5. Remove from heat, allow to cool down, add avocado, and blend until smooth. Refrigerate until ready to serve.
6. In the meantime, steam asparagus tips until tender. Do not overcook.
7. Remove the soup from the fridge, add lemon juice, and stir well.
8. Sprinkle with tarragon, black pepper, a dollop of yogurt, and asparagus tips, and serve.

As we wrap up our exploration of soups, let's enjoy the delicious smell that fills your kitchen. These recipes have been more than just meals – they've been about feeling better. And each recipe is like a big hug for your gut. Remember the cozy feeling you get from a good bowl of soup, and let that feeling stay with you as you enjoy each spoonful. Carry this comforting experience with you, and let these soups become a part of your journey to feeling your best.

6
Conclusion

We are at the end of our culinary adventure. Its mission was to invigorate our bodies as we age, ease menopause symptoms, elevate energy levels, and help our weight loss, using the power of whole foods. Throughout this journey together, we've discovered the fascinating world of nutrition and explored the profound impact nourishing foods can have on our bodies. And we used smoothies, salads, and soups as powerful and delightful instruments for achieving our health goals.

From the very beginning, my goal was to provide you with practical, simple yet delicious recipes, as actionable steps to transform your health. As you continue your quest for better health, I encourage you to use these recipes as a road map to making healthier choices, improving your eating habits, and building a better connection with your body. Take the initiative and opt for nourishing foods and say "no" to gut offenders.

Experiment with your own ideas, create your own recipes with the ingredients that speak to you. And make conscious choices about what you eat. Remember that every ingredient you choose is a step towards enhancing your well-being.

I want to thank you for joining me on this journey. It's been a true privilege to share my knowledge, experience, and passion with you.

Your commitment to your health is inspiring to me, and I hope the knowledge you've gained here continues to inspire you, too. As we say goodbye, I believe you will continue to flourish on this path to better health.

Will You Light the Path to Better Health for More Women?

Thank you for purchasing my book and taking the time to read it. Your insights and feedback are invaluable to me. Please reach out and share your experience with the recipes, I'd love to learn what you're cooking in your kitchen!

If you've enjoyed this book and found value in its pages, please share your reflections by offering a review on Amazon. Your honest review can play a vital role in helping other women discover the transformative potential of these recipes, enabling them to embark on their own path to menopause vitality. Thank you for helping me help them!

To leave a review on Amazon, please follow this link **https://www.amazon.com/dp/B0CHGQP6D5#customerReviews** or scan the QR Code below. Thank you!

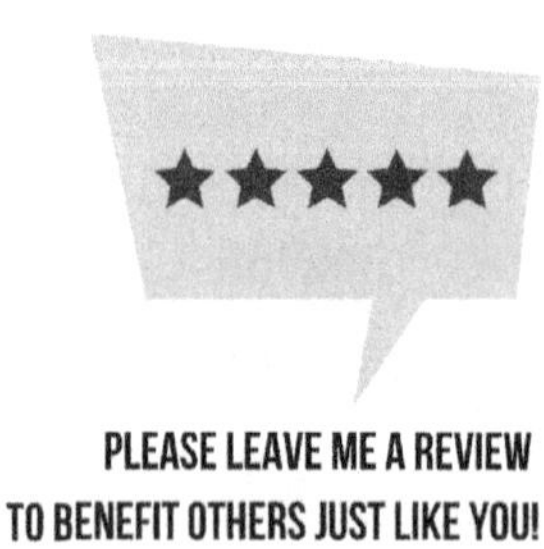
★★★★★
PLEASE LEAVE ME A REVIEW
TO BENEFIT OTHERS JUST LIKE YOU!

About the Author

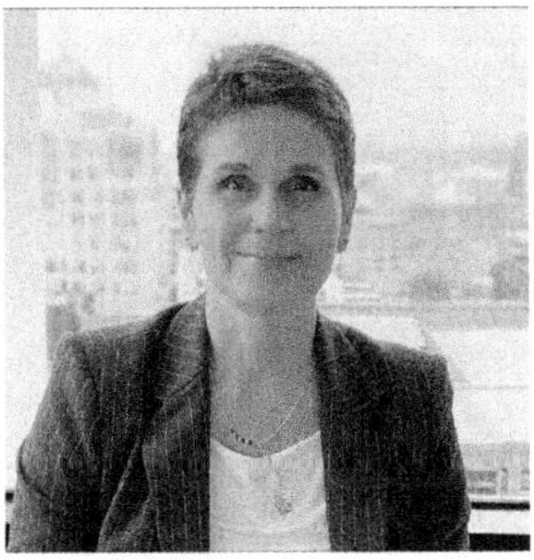

Lara West is a health and wellness advocate dedicated to empowering readers through her insightful writings. With a particular emphasis on women's and midlife health, Lara shares relatable and practical tips drawn from her personal experiences that deeply resonate with her readers.

Her journey began in her mid-forties as she faced perimenopausal symptoms, leaky gut syndrome, an autoimmune disease, and the challenges of caregiving for a family member with dementia. This transformative period ignited her passion for understanding gut health and its significant impact on overall well-being, as well as the importance of self-care for caregivers.

Lara's commitment to holistic wellness inspires her to share practical strategies for navigating the challenges of middle age, caregiving, and maintaining an active lifestyle. She emphasizes the importance of self-care and balanced living, passionately advocating for an active and fulfilling life in retirement, ensuring the best years are ahead. Lara encourages readers to reclaim their vitality and joy at every stage of life.

Through her clear and structured writing style, infused with compassion and relatability, Lara makes complex health topics accessible and engaging, inspiring others to take charge of their health and well-being.

You can reach Lara via her website https://larawestbooks.com or Amazon Author Page https://www.amazon.com/stores/Lara-West/author/B0BV3F1YK7

LaraWestBooks.com

Amazon Author Page

Also by Lara West

1. "The Great Retirement Escape: Your Guide to Journeys Across the Globe, Adventures Close to Home, Inspiring Outdoor Activities, and Fun Active Lifestyle for Your Best Years Yet"

2. "Retirement Reinvented: Your Inspiring Guide to Creative Expression, Intellectual Growth, Entrepreneurial Ventures, and Leaving a Legacy for a Fulfilling and Meaningful Life After Work"

3. "7 Healthy Gut Habits For Women Over 40: Get Your Life Back Using Intermittent Fasting, Nutrition, and Self-Care to Restore Gut Microbiome for Weight Loss and Increased Energy"

4. "5 Pathways to Vagus Nerve Mastery for Women Over 40: Holistic Methods to Reduce Anxiety, Clear Brain Fog, Improve Gut Health, and Balance Weight During Perimenopause and" Menopause

5. "Gut Health Made Easy for Women over 40: Recipes to Revitalize Your Body and Mind, Manage Menopause Symptoms, Balance Hormones, and Lose Weight with Delicious Smoothies, Salads, and Soups"

6. "Joyful Transition For Women Over 40: Finding Gratitude and

Thriving in Menopause with Empowering Affirmations, Journaling, and Positive Mindset Practices"

7. "The Ultimate Gut Health Collection for Women Over 40: Reclaim Your Vitality, Lose Weight, and Manage Menopause Symptoms with Intermittent Fasting, Self-Care, Balanced Nutrition, and Delicious Recipes"
8. "The Ultimate Mind-Body Harmony Collection for Women over 40: Reduce Anxiety, Clear Brain Fog, Improve Gut Health, and Thrive in Menopause with Vagus Nerve Mastery and Positive Mindset Practices"
9. "The Self-Care Guide for Dementia Caregivers: Proven Practices to Reduce Stress, Overcome Burnout, and Find Balance and Joy in the Caregiving Journey"

References

1. The Health Benefits of Dietary Fibre. Thomas M. Barber, Stefan Kabisch, Andreas F. H. Pfeiffer, and Martin O. Weickert. Published online 2020 Oct 21. https://www.ncbi.nlm.nih.gov/pmc/articles/PMC7589116/

2. 22 High Fiber Foods You Should Eat. https://www.healthline.com/nutrition/22-high-fiber-foods

3. Effect of Gluten-Free Diet on Gut Microbiota Composition in Patients with Celiac Disease and Non-Celiac Gluten/Wheat Sensitivity. Giacomo Caio, Lisa Lungaro, Nicola Segata, Matteo Guarino, Giorgio Zoli, Umberto Volta,5, and Roberto De Gior gio.Published online 2020 Jun 19. https://www.ncbi.nlm.nih.gov/pmc/articles/PMC7353361/

4. The Importance of Prebiotics. November 15, 2022. https://www.lifespan.org/lifespan-living/importance-prebiotics

5. Fermented Foods for Gut Health. OCTOBER 2019. Barbara Olendzkikelly Sanders. UMass Chan Medical School, Center for Applied Nutrition; https://www.umassmed.edu/nutrition/blog/blog-posts/2019/6/fermented-foods-for-gut-health/

6. Impact of Omega-3 Fatty Acids on the Gut Microbiota. Published online 2017 Dec 7. Lara Costantini, Romina Molinari,

Barbara Farinon, and Nicolò Merendino. https://www.ncbi.nlm.nih.gov/pmc/articles/PMC5751248/

7. Omega-3 for your Health. By Linda Rath | Updated Dec. 8, 2022 https://www.arthritis.org/health-wellness/treatment/complementary-therapies/supplements-and-vitamins/omega-3-fatty-acids-for-health
8. The complete guide to omega-3-rich foods. Medical News Today. Last medically reviewed on June 30, 2022https://www.medicalnewstoday.com/articles/323144
9. Gut Microbiota and Inflammation. Published online 2011. Asa Hakansson and Goran Molin. https://www.ncbi.nlm.nih.gov/pmc/articles/PMC3257638/
10. Anti-Inflammatory Foods and Foods that Cause Inflammation. Author: Stephen Devries, MD. Gaples Institute. https://www.gaplesinstitute.org/anti-inflammatory-foods-and-foods-that-cause-inflammation/
11. Vitamin A and Carotenoids. National Institutes of Health. https://ods.od.nih.gov/factsheets/VitaminA-Consumer/
12. Vitamin D. Fact Sheet for Health Professionals. National Institutes of Health. od.nih.gov/factsheets/VitaminD-HealthProfessionals
13. Vitamin E, the Nutrition Source. Harvard School of Public Health. https://www.hsph.harvard.edu/nutritionsource/vitamin-e/
14. Why Is Vitamin B Complex Important, and Where Do I Get It? https://www.healthline.com/health/food-nutrition/vitamin-b-complex

15. Zinc Benefits Every Woman Should Know About. BY KAYLA BLANTON AND CHRISTINE BYRNE. Published: AUG 29, 2023 https://www.womenshealthmag.com/food/g19967379/signs-youre-not-getting-zinc/

16. 6 Reasons Women Need Magensium. Health Central. https://www.healthcentral.com/slideshow/6-reasons-women-need-magnesium

17. 7 Science-Based Health Benefits of Selenium. HealthLine. By Jillian Kubala MS, RD. https://www.healthline.com/nutrition/selenium-benefits

18. What Does Potassium Do for Your Body? A Detailed Review. By Ryan Raman. https://www.healthline.com/nutrition/what-does-potassium-do

19. Benefits and sources of calcium. Medical News Today. Medically reviewed by Kathy W. Warwick, R.D., CDE, Nutrition — By Peter Morales-Brown — Updated on June 27, 2023. https://www.medicalnewstoday.com/articles/248958

20. Top Benefits of Vitamin K. Cleveland Clinic. https://health.clevelandclinic.org/vitamin-k/

21. Sprouts: Are They Good for You? Written by WebMD Editorial Contributors. Medically Reviewed by Jabeen Begum, MD on September 21, 2022 https://www.webmd.com/diet/sprouts-good-for-you

22. Superfood Powder Benefits. https://www.mybrightcore.com/blogs/articles/superfood-powder-benefits

23. 9 Important Functions of Protein in Your Body. By Gavin Van De Walle, MS, RD — Updated on February 15, 2023 https://w

ww.healthline.com/nutrition/functions-of-protein

24. How does dairy affect gut health? Aaqeelah Floris; 01 September 2021 https://www.lifehealthcare.co.za/news-and-info-hub/latest-news/how-does-dairy-affect-gut-health/

25. Excessive consumption of red meat can change gut microbiota, leading to the appearance of heart disease. https://www.gutmicrobiotaforhealth.com/excessive-consumption-of-red-meat-can-change-gut-microbiota-leading-to-the-appearance-of-heart-disease

26. Best Foods to Balance Hormones. BY CHRISTINE TRAXLER, MD. https://zayacare.com/blog/best-foods-to-balance-hormones/

27. Health Benefits of Mushrooms. Medically Reviewed by Jabeen Begum, MD on September 08, 2023 Written by WebMD Editorial Contributor. https://www.webmd.com/diet/health-benefits-mushrooms

28. 10 Fresh Herbs with Great Health Benefits. https://www.aarp.org/health/healthy-living/info-2022/fresh-herb-health-benefits.html

29. Why Smoothies Are a More Gut-Healthy Choice Than Juice, According to a Gastroenterologist. By Karla Walsh. https://www.eatingwell.com/article/8024320/smoothie-more-gut-healthy-than-juice-gastroenterologist/

30. How a Soup Cleanse Can Heal Your Gut. https://detoxkitchen.co.uk/health/how-a-soup-cleanse-can-heal-your-gut

Printed in Dunstable, United Kingdom

68265900R00090